The following excerpts from various news media over the past 44 years illustrate the concept and research direction that is presented and expanded in *Why Arthritis?*

Dr. Brown Discloses Rheumatic Research
RADICALLY NEW evidence that rheumatic diseases may be due to an unusual type of microbe has been offered for the first time as a result of the research by Dr. Thomas McPherson Brown and associates.

—The George Washington University Record
June 13, 1951

Hope Held Out for Cure of Rheumatic Ills
Washington Research Team Announces New Concept on Causes and Cure. (Story reported in hundreds of newspapers across the U.S.A.)

—Associated Press
June 8, 1951

New Arthritis Theory Told at Medical Parley
—Globe
Boston, Mass.
June 8, 1951

GWU Doctor's 'New Concept' Reported Effective in Arthritis
A bold, new concept of the cause and course of rheumatic diseases, and a new and effective treatment developed were reported.

—Washington Post
June 9, 1951

Medical Researcher Isolates Crippler Germs, Believe to be the Cause of Arthritis
—International News Service
June 9, 1951

Science in Review—For Rheumatic Ills
Antibiotics are found helpful with or without cortisone.

—New York Times, Editorial
June 9, 1951

i

Revolt Against Indifference Spurred Study of Rheumatics
"The story behind the development of a hopeful new concept of the cause and treatment of rheumatic diseases is the story of a Washington doctor's revolt against medical indifference and trial-by-error methods."

—Washington Post
June 10, 1951

Contra el Rheuma
Nueva esperanza de curacion.

—Vision (Spanish)
June 12, 1951

Medicine—Rheumatic Disease Hope
Terramycin and albumin may be remedies for rheumatic disease. Basis for treatment is new-old theory that disease is germ caused.

—Science News Letter
June 16, 1951

Arthritis Research: A New Approach
—Pathfinder
Philadelphia, PA
June 27, 1951

Pfizer Announces Special Terramycin. Antibiotics Attack Organism held to Cause Rheumatic Ills
"Special dosage forms of terramycin intended especially for clinical research in the treatment of arthritis."

—Drug Trade News
New York, N.Y.
July 8, 1951

Germ or Deficiency?
—Newsweek
July 9, 1951

"A totally different theory as to the cause of rheumatism and arthritis has been propounded. It means, if true, that such

ii

diseases can really be cured".
> —*Business Week (McGraw Hill)*
> *July 14, 1951*

Effective Treatment for Rheumatic Diseases is Reported
> —*Science Air Bulletin*
> *July 18, 1951*

Science and the Citizen: Arthritis Germs?
Described new concept as "one of the most exciting leads."
> —*Scientific American*
> *August, 1951*

Arthritis—Full scale article calls new concept
"by far the most significant and hopeful new development"
> —*Good Housekeeping*
> *by Maxine Davis*
> *August, 1951*

New Approach to Treatment of Arthritis
> —*Nursing World*
> *August, 1951*

New basic theory about arthritis, developed by GWU research team selected as one of the top 10 biggest science stories in 1951
> —*Popular Science,*
> *December, 1951*

The Arthritis Story, 1948-1968 The beginning - Early years
> —*G.W.*
> *The George Washing Univ. Magazine*
> *Spring 1968*

Mycoplasma Approach to Arthritis Holds Cure Possibility
> —*Drug Research Reports, 1969*

Arthritis Test with a Gorilla Found Hopeful
> —*Medical Tribune & Medical News*
> *World Wide Report*
> *November, 20, 1969*

iii

Mycoplasmas in Arthritis & Urethritis—Editorial
—*J.A.M.A.*
January, 1974

Scientist Cites Mycoplasmas as the Cause of Rheumatoid Arthritis
—*Rapid City Journal, S.D.*
September, 1980

Success with Gorillas Yields High Hopes for Humans
Once crippled with arthritis, Tomoka is energetic, healthy.
—*Miami Herald*
U.P. International
June, 1981

New Hope for Arthritis Sufferers?
Paris — Great hope for sufferers from crippling arthritis, through administration of properly spaced tetracycline combined with anti-inflammatory agents, is being held out here by an internationally recognized rheumatologist..
—*Decatur Daily (Alabama)*
June 28, 1981

Drug treatment offers hope of Arthritis Cure for Millions
"An antibiotic has brought amazing results in 35 severe rheumatoid arthritis patients".
—*Star*
July 14, 1981

Primate Therapy Stirs Controversy
Physicians Question Gorilla Tactics in War on Arthritis.
—*Washington Star*
by Patrice Gaines-Carter
July 26, 1981

Gorilla's Arthritis Cure Gives New Hope to Millions
—*Globe*
by Penny Jacobs
Sept. 15, 1981

Rheuma - den Ursachen Naher?
Fur Gorillas Antiphlogistika mit tetracyclinen.
—Selecta 47 (German)
23 Nov. 1981

Patients Rally 'Round Maverick Arthritis Doctor
"For years Dr. Brown and his associate Dr. Harold Clark have been zeroing in on a viral-like agent called mycoplasma, the known cause of rheumatoid arthritis in animals."
—Alexandria Journal, VA
November 1982

Mycoplasmas and Human Arthritis
—Arthritis Literature News - 1983

"The cause of rheumatoid arthritis is still unknown and its treatment is very unsatisfactory."
—National Institutes of Health, 1983

"We must take seriously the possibility that mycoplasmas cause arthritis in humans."
—National Arthritis Advisory Board, 1984

"We have no predictably efficacious therapy for rheumatoid arthritis at the present time."
—National Arthritis Advisory Board, 1984

The Arthritis—Infection Connection: Skeptics Reconsider
One rheumatologist who's convinced that Mycoplasma plays a major role in rheumatoid arthritis is Dr. T. McP. Brown - who has treated more than 10,000 RA patients with extended regimens of antibiotics for almost 40 years.
—Medical World News (Cover Story)
by Mark L. Fuerst
September 9, 1985

"Some rheumatologists have long advocated tetracycline antibiotic as an appropriate treatment for rheumatoid arthritis."
—National Institutes of Health, 1991

Gold Salts Not Effective, Arthritis Study Says

—Tampa Tribune (AP)
March, 1991

Arthritis—Learning to Live With It
Now there is renewed interest in their (tetracycline treatment devised by the late rheumatologist Dr. Thomas McPherson Brown) possible usefulness as a treatment for arthritis in people.

—Washington Post - Health
by Sandy Rovner
June 15, 1991

"In 1988, researcher Thomas McPherson Brown, M.D., presented a study showing that minocycline was effective in the treatment of rheumatoid arthritis."

—American College of Rheumatology, 1993

Patient Information - A New Decade of Hope
Antibiotics (minocycline) for rheumatoid arthritis. Investigators concluded that minocycline was effective for treatment of rheumatoid arthritis.

—Editors, American College of Rheumatology
November 16, 1993

Minocycline Therapy Looks Promising Against Rheumatoid Arthritis

—Family Practice news
February 1, 1994

Researchers Find Acne Drug (minocycline) Can Soothe Rheumatoid Arthritis Pain
"Patients who suffer from mild to moderate rheumatoid arthritis now have the choice of another therapeutic agent."

—Associated Press Report
January 15, 1995

Study Backs Antibiotic as Arthritis Aid
"Antibiotic treatment for RA, a therapy widely discredited after its heyday in the 1960s and '70s, now turns out to work—perhaps as

vi

well as current treatments for the mysterious crippling disease."

"The cause of RA is one of medicine's major puzzles. Ironically the NIAMSD has opposed a thorough test of antibiotic therapy for arthritis. It relented only under steady lobbying from advocates of the unorthodox treatment. Dr. Brown, who died in 1989, believed that arthritis was caused by an organism called mycoplasma."

—*The Boston Globe*
by Richard A. Knox
January 15, 1995

"Could tomorrow's Best Treatment for RA be a drug or drugs that exist Today?"

—*Arthritis Today (AP)*
July 8, 1995

Newspaper Clippings

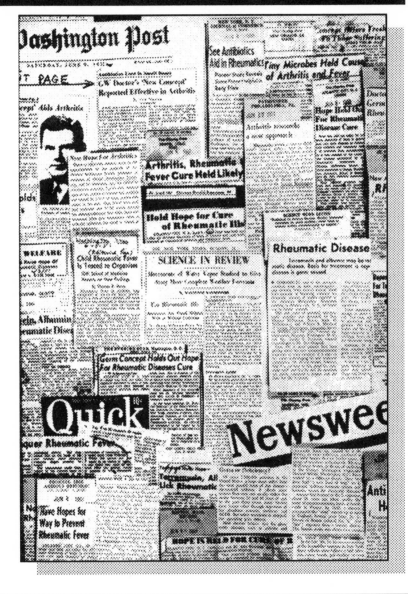

WHY ARTHRITIS?

SEARCHING FOR THE CAUSE AND THE CURE

OF RHEUMATOID DISEASE

Harold W. Clark, Ph.D.

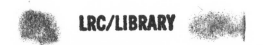

Cover design by Dunn + Associates
Edited by Karen L. Jacob
Typeset by New Images
Printed in the United States of America

Grateful acknowledgment is made to the Egyptian Museum, Cairo, Egypt, and the Metropolitan Museum of Art, New York City, New York, for permission to reprint museum art reproductions.

Publisher's Cataloging in Publication
(Prepared by Quality Books, Inc.)

Clark, Harold W.
    Why Arthritis? searching for the cause and the cure of rheumatoid disease/by Harold W. Clark, Ph.D.
    p. cm
    Includes bibliographical references and index.
    LCCN 95-80337
    ISBN   0-936417-51-X

    1. Arthritis.   I. Title

RC633.C53 1996   616.7'22
                             QB195-20542

This Book is Dedicated:

To my dear wife and children for their indulgence and sharing in my dream.

To the staff and trustees of the Arthritis Institute,[1] especially Rachael, Jack, Irene, and Jackie for their many years of loyal support, without whom this book could not have been written.

To the late Thomas McPherson Brown, with whom I had the pleasure of working for 35 years and the opportunity to share in the often controversial search for the mycoplasma cause and tetracycline cure of rheumatoid diseases.

To the patients, volunteers, and friends of the Arthritis Institute and especially those at the National Hospital who contributed many dollars and hours of essential support and encouragement.

To the veterinarians and zoo staffs around the world, especially at the National Zoological Park in Washington, DC, who generously provided their time and great interest in helping to solve the arthritis problem.

To the Mycoplasma Research Institute[2] for its encouragement and full support of the book's preparation.

---

[1]   The Arthritis Institute of the National Hospital in Arlington, VA, has been renamed the Thomas McPherson Brown Arthritis Institute in memory of its founder and former director.

[2]   The Mycoplasma Research Institute, a nonprofit corporation committed to the promotion of research and education toward understanding mycoplasma diseases, was established by Harold W. Clark, Ph.D.

Talk With Your Doctor

This book is not intended as a substitute for the medical advice of your physician. Readers should talk with a practicing physician concerning their personal health and particularly about any unusual symptoms that may require medical attention. The opinions expressed are those of the authors and do not necessarily represent those of others presented in other publications.

TABLE OF CONTENTS

PREFACE

Why Arthritis? provides readers with the all-important ingredient of hope that is essential for a healthy and pain-free future. The author describes the little-known research efforts behind the most effective and safest antibiotic treatment of rheumatoid arthritis that has been just recently recognized. The book documents the controversial paths taken by medical experts who failed to find the cure or the cause of rheumatoid arthritis.

The readers will learn why the medical establishment has taken over 40 years to test and recognize a safe and effective antibiotic treatment. Even though some atypical infectious agent has long been suspected to be the cause of rheumatoid arthritis, only one doctor persisted in developing and testing beneficial antibiotic treatment—renowned rheumatologist Thomas McPherson Brown, M.D., my close associate for 40 years.

The arthritic or rheumatoid disorders have remained a mystery for centuries as the search for the causes and cures continued to elude scientists. The word arthritis continues to be used broadly to include the hundreds of systemic rheumatoid disorders that can have both joint and multiple tissue symptoms. Unlike other books that describe the variety of symptoms and the temporary band-aid therapy, the author pursues the therapeutic elimination of the causative agent(s) and not just the palliation of resulting symptoms.

The book explains and provides a critical analysis of why it has taken the medical establishment 40 years to test and recognize antibiotic treatment as the safest and most effective rheumatoid arthritis therapy. The book documents reports from the National Institutes of Health, the Arthritis Foundation, the American Rheumatology Association, and the U.S. Congress, which have provided the research direction and are responsible for the leadership and financial research support.

The book documents and describes the various circumstances, events, people, and organizations that have influenced the course of arthritis research over the past 45 years. It answers both the patients' and doctors' questions about why the cure and the cause have not been found and why it has taken so long to recognize a safe and effective antibiotic treatment as first reported in the 7th National Arthritis Congress.

In view of the unsatisfactory and failing results of the currently available therapies, the beneficial results from recent hope for a pain-free future. The report of the clinical results stated that: "Not only did the antibiotics significantly reduce symptoms, but side effects were minimal and less severe than observed for most other common rheumatoid arthritis treatments."

The readers will be pleased to learn that a safe and beneficial treatment for rheumatoid arthritis is now available and at a much lower cost. They will also learn about the pioneering efforts and struggle of a leading investigator to develop the antibiotic treatment that has brought researchers much closer to understanding the infectious cause. Informing patients about the politics and competitive actions limiting research progress will enable them to better understand the many years of being told that the cause and cure of rheumatoid arthritis were unknown.

Unlike other books, the author reviews the many problems that researchers face in seeking the cure and the cause of arthritis. The story of tetracycline's role in rheumatoid arthritis could be comparable to the development, testing, and acceptance of other wonder drugs, such as cortisone, penicillin, and insulin. To help patients better understand their disease and treatment, the author describes the research directions that have finally resulted in an effective treatment of rheumatoid arthritis, the most costly and crippling medical disorder. Finding an effective control of rheumatoid arthritis will lead to its prevention and thus save billions of dollars for research on other chronic diseases.

H.W.C.

INTRODUCTION

"It is a distressing fact of life that although there are drugs to relieve the pain and reduce the inflammation of arthritis, there are no cures for most of the more than 100 types of this painful and sometimes crippling disease. . . Not only are there few cures, but also scientists don't know for sure what causes most types of the disease" (FDA, 1993).

Arthritis comes in many different forms or types classified according to symptomatology, which does not exclude common causes and cures for the different types. Osteoarthritis or degenerative joint disease is the most prevalent form of arthritis, increasing with age as the joints undergo degeneration from wear and tear and other unknown causes. *Why Arthritis?* primarily asks what causes the rheumatoid diseases, such as the chronic inflammatory connective tissues of rheumatoid arthritis, and the collagen vascular disorders, such as Lupus, and what therapy controls or cures them.

Many books have been written to help arthritis patients understand their symptoms and treatments so that they can better cope and live with their disease. Unlike other books that describe what is known about arthritis and what patients should or should not do, this book takes a look at why research has not found the cause and cure for arthritis and what the future will bring. Reviewing some of the research directions taken over the past 50 years leads one to question the present conclusion that the cause and cure for rheumatoid diseases are not yet known but scientists have discovered some promising leads. What are these promising leads, and is anyone exploring them? Why do researchers continue to fall short of the goal? If infectious agents are the promising lead or suspected cause, why haven't they been identified? How much progress has been made toward understanding the cause and cure, and will the 21st century bring answers or more promises?

Arthritis patients want to know all about their disease, especially why they have arthritis and why it costs so much. Patients can take only small comfort in knowing that medical researchers are making progress in understanding their illness when one costly drug after another fails them. Patients are discouraged by being constantly told that the cause and cure are not known and they should learn to live with their arthritis.

The primary aim of this book is to improve the treatment of arthritis patients by helping them better understand the successes and failures in searching for the causes and cures. Significant information already exists that should provide patients with hope and encouragement. Other basic research findings have led to our currently accepted concepts and knowledge about the causes of the disease processes and how medications, like aspirin, stop the symptoms, pain, and inflammation without stopping the disease progression.

The technical advances to measure arthritis symptoms have far outpaced safe and effective therapeutic control of symptoms. Aspirin, an age-old remedy, is still the number one drug of choice. We now know that daily aspirin may also delay or reduce cardiovascular diseases, which can also develop in a variety of arthritic disorders from damage to kidneys, lungs, and neurologic systems, as well as the heart and blood vessels, resulting in decreased longevity.

A story in *The New York Times* noted in 1985 that "rough estimates by a Congressional Survey suggests that Americans waste nearly two billion dollars a year on quack remedies for arthritis." In view of the increasing number of approved drug failures and other stopgap palliative therapies, it appears that the disease is only temporarily delayed at a far greater cost. Perhaps Congress should also investigate the waste and huge profits made on the ineffective therapies already approved by the Food and Drug Administration.

Determining which drug therapy is safe and effective for each patient is always difficult. Although we have very similar chemical or metabolic blueprints, subtle differences reflect our unique fingerprints or genetic makeup. Molecular, biological, and genetic researchers are identifying certain differences that appear to contribute to an individual's susceptibility or predisposition to developing specific diseases. Even where the causative agent and disease mechanism are similar, physiological differences between the young and the elderly of both sexes can further contribute to the unique display of symptomatic or pathogenic expressions in each arthritis patient and each patient's response to drug treatment.

Patients whose drug treatments continue to fail and who face taking stronger and more toxic medications want to know what's next and why the so-called proven remedies do not help them. They start shopping for safe and effective alternative treatments outside accepted medical practice, especially when rheumatoid arthritis has become the most costly disease to treat. This book takes an in-depth tour of a promising alternative approach to arthritis treatment developed and first used by the Arthritis Institute staff in 1948. Tetracycline therapy has been used successfully to control the disease mechanisms and eliminate a suspected cause of rheumatoid arthritis.

Perhaps the greatest stimulant prompting this review of arthritis research efforts came when our NIH grant application for support of a clinical trial with tetracycline was disapproved in 1984. A noted rheumatologist on the peer-review committee stated, "What are you guys trying to do, put us out of business?" If our research efforts and accomplishments were all that threatening, perhaps the public should have a chance to review them with the hope that they will help to eliminate and prevent the most costly and crippling rheumatoid diseases. A medical director of the Arthritis Foundation told one of our patients that if our research efforts were proven to be right, we should receive a Nobel Prize.

Efforts to demonstrate the effectiveness of tetracycline therapy were initiated and first reported over 40 years ago by Thomas McPherson Brown. Ironically, only two weeks after his untimely death in 1989, NIH requested grant applications for the controlled clinical trials of tetracycline therapy in rheumatoid arthritis that he had been seeking. When the results become known, doctors and some 400 million arthritis patients around the world will want to know why tetracycline treatment has been ignored by the medical establishment for so long. In fact, the preliminary results of the clinical trials were so promising that NIH requested grant applications for studies of mycoplasmas and other infectious agents as a cause for rheumatoid diseases in 1993 and a pilot study for intravenous antibiotics for rheumatoid arthritis in 1994. Hopefully these studies will also lead to the control and prevention of many other unsolved chronic diseases that have similar causative mechanisms.

During the past 40 years, many patients visited our research facilities to learn more about their rheumatoid disorders, laboratory tests, and medications. How does wear and tear or old age cause osteoarthritis in some people? Do people who talk a lot or chew gum develop arthritic jaws or temporomandibular joint (TMJ) syndrome? What causes pain, swelling, early morning stiffness, fatigue, and depression? Does replacing joints, organs, or clogged blood vessels eliminate the cause of their disease, or are these also palliative and high-cost band aids? Providing patients with this additional information has helped them to evaluate their own situation as well as new information and claims they learn about in the news media. Understanding what they see and hear makes the patients better equipped to manage their disease.

Patients often wonder why they have arthritis or other rheumatoid disorders. Was it an infection? Was it inevitable, or could something have been done to avoid or prevent it? What can be done to help lessen or stop the disease? Will my children inherit the disease, or will I transmit it to them? A recent front page article in the *St. Petersburg Times* reported that osteoarthritis is caused by a genetic disorder in certain families.[1] Does that mean it is not caused by aging or wear and tear as previously reported and will be inherited? Or is the genetic abnormality caused by the disease?

Although much of the available information is still fragmented and often controversial, a better understanding of the complex-

---

[1]   Based on a Proceedings of the National Academy of Sciences, USA, report in September 1990.

ities of rheumatoid disorders should facilitate and encourage better communication between patients and doctors that is often hampered by the highly specialized language of scientific research. Telling people about both the positive and negative research findings in lay terms provides the all-important therapeutic ingredient of hope, which is not provided by only telling them that the causes and cures have not been found but soon will be.

The following chapters will review and explore past and current research efforts to find answers to the many perplexing questions about arthritis that have been left unanswered. High-risk or predisposing factors, suspected and probable causes, the role of animal models, and the search for a magic bullet as well as the infectious cause will be discussed. This information should provide a better picture of what is on the horizon.

If we are going to solve the many chronic diseases of unknown origins, medicine must become a full science and not just an art as Lewis Thomas suggested in his book *The Youngest Science: Notes of a Medicine Watcher.* Both sides of the equation or reaction, the patient and the doctor, must be known and knowledgeable. The more that patients know about the physiology and chemistry of their disease, the better they will understand and be able to help doctors measure and determine cause and effect relationships of what is going on inside their minds as well as their bodies. What patients believe can have an enormous effect on their physical health, especially if they have accepted an inevitable and incurable disease. This knowledge is especially important because patients can think and worry about their disease and unpaid medical bills as well as tell, record, and show where it hurts. Unfortunately, patients are also exposed to half-baked commercials and other media hype promoting the latest beneficial nutrients and extra-strength arthritis therapy, which greatly adds to their despair and financial burden.

WHY ARTHRITIS?

SEARCHING FOR THE CAUSE AND THE CURE

OF RHEUMATOID DISEASE

Chapter I
What Is Arthritis?

To solve a problem, one must first define the problem. Learning all you can about your crippling disease and available therapy, even when there are no known cause and cure, helps to remove the barriers of fear and guilt about being sick that can be more disabling than the disease itself. Learning to cope and live with your disease should not provide a sense of defeat and loss of hope. Cope but don't capitulate.

In searching for the cause and cure, it is essential to know exactly what problem is to be solved. The range of arthritis-associated diseases are far too broad for anyone to research or discuss and for starters the study must be limited to one class, such as diffuse connective tissue diseases and rheumatoid arthritis. Another separate class is osteoarthritis or degenerative joint disease, the most prevalent form of arthritis, increasing with age and the joints under degeneration from unknown cause. It differs primarily from the other chronic rheumatoid diseases by the absence of immunologic and inflammatory responses. A brief explanation of some medical terminology used in this book is provided below.

Arthritis is a vague descriptive term derived from the Greek word *arthro* meaning joint and the suffix *itis* meaning inflammation. It is commonly used to denote discomfort or abnormal joints. People with arthritis have a pretty good idea of what constitutes a

3

joint: two opposing bones lined by hard cartilaginous material surrounded by synovial tissue. The bones are hinged together by connective and muscle tissues and controlled by tendons and nerves, all of which are fed by a vascular blood supply. Inflammation is another very broad descriptive term that is difficult to describe as it has many causes and can apply to any tissue that has a blood supply. In appearance, this can be a warm, reddish, swollen, tender, or painful area of the skin surrounding a stiff joint. Unless otherwise demonstrated, the symptoms are assumed to derive from an underlying tissue, such as the synovium, referred to as synovitis, or inflamed synovial tissue. Other inflamed tissues surrounding a particular joint are referred to as tendonitis (tendon), bursitis (bursa), myositis (muscle), neuritis (nerve), and vasculitis (blood vessel). Although it is possible to have an arthritic joint without inflammation, such as reported in the more common osteoarthritis (degenerative joint disease), it is less likely because an irritated joint usually results in some form of inflammation.

Searching for the initial causes and sequence of events remains the major problem. If an irritated joint results in inflammation, then what causes the irritation? Usually the introduction of any foreign or altered native substance, such as micro-organisms, chemical and inert particles, or physical trauma to a joint is enough of an irritant to initiate arthritis. The resulting arthritis comes and goes in many different forms and intensities that are highly influenced by the production and control of biological mediators of inflammation are response to an irritant. The magnitude and duration of inflammation are influenced by the extent of tissue injury. An irritant also may cause a mildly deformed joint with no signs of inflammation. Inflammation around a joint space that looks and feels normal can be detected using a highly sensitive radioisotopic scan or the more costly magnet resonance imaging (MRI). In 1978, our clinic reported the successful use of the radioisotope scan technique to measure the reduction of inflammation in RA patients treated with tetracycline.

Rheumatoid Diseases

The real problem that researchers must solve comes when the inflammation persists and none of the suspected agents or conditions can be identified and related to the resulting symptoms. A causative agent has been identified in various forms of arthritis: uric acid crystals in gout, bacteria or viruses in septic or reactive arthritis, or a sprain resulting in traumatic arthritis. But what agents are causing the hundreds of other chronic forms of arthritis and related rheumatoid diseases? Perhaps the agents have come and gone or are residing in some distant tissues. In searching for the causative agents, perhaps researchers have been looking in the wrong place, at the wrong time, and for the wrong reasons.

Arthritis is often used interchangeably or collectively with the term rheumatism, which is derived from the Greek word *rheuma*, meaning a mucous or watery discharge. It is used to describe joint and muscle symptoms of unknown or unexplained causes. However, rheumatic fever, displaying arthritis, heart disease, pleural fluid, and fever in children, is known to be caused by a streptococcal bacterium and is often controlled by penicillin therapy.

Today, several medical societies, associations, and nonprofit foundations are committed to the study and control of the various forms of arthritis. The national medical society of rheumatologists who specialize in arthritis is now called the American College of Rheumatology (ACR), formerly the American Rheumatism Association, Inc. (ARA).[1] They publish the medical journal *Arthritis and Rheumatism,* which covers both the known and unknown causes of arthritis. The other health professionals—nurses, physical therapists, occupational therapists, and social workers—who comprise the Allied Health Professions Association (AHPA) are important members of research teams. The Arthritis Foundation (AF), the largest non-profit group committed to promoting support for those with the disease, was organized in 1948[2].

Although the term arthritis is more encompassing it is less appropriate than the term rheumatoid diseases because other tissues and organs are involved than just joints, so in the search for the

---

[1] Organized in 1934 as the American Association for the Study and Control of Rheumatic Diseases, the ARA merged with the Arthritis Foundation as its medical section and later became a separate organization.

[2] It was originally known as the Arthritis and Rheumatism Foundation but renamed after a split from the National Polio Foundation, which also supports research on crippling diseases in children.

causes anatomical areas must be considered. For a description of relevant medical terminology and a review of the various forms of arthritis, basic disease mechanisms, clinical symptoms, and treatment, see the latest *Primer on the Rheumatic Diseases* published by the Arthritis Foundation. Written primarily for doctors and allied health professionals, the average patient may find it complex and difficult to understand. If not, it can be used as a basis for discussion with a doctor or therapist. In the 1993 edition, the primer stated in the discussion on scleroderma, or progressive systematic sclerosis (PSS), that a dramatic clinical improvement was noted after tetracycline therapy (although the causes of PSS are unknown). There is no explanation why antibiotic therapy was used or any mention of tetracycline's anti-inflammatory and anticollagenase properties.

Osteoarthritis, or degenerative joint disease, the most common form of arthritis, was once thought to be an inevitable disease of old age caused by wear and tear. The cause or initiating event leading to this chronic progressive disorder remains unknown.

More appropriate descriptive terms of the rheumatoid disorders have been used, which reflect our increasing knowledge of the disease mechanisms or target tissues and not just the symptoms. These include collagen vascular, connective tissue, autoimmune, and immune complex disorders. The search has narrowed from nonspecific arthritis to rheumatism to specific diseases or tissue mechanisms of unknown causes.

Many different causes of rheumatoid diseases have been suggested and pursued. Upon further study and review, researchers may find that a common agent and mechanism can cause various symptoms in tissues because of differences between individual patients. For example, because of the many associative factors (age, sex, genetics, and history), a microorganism could cause rheumatoid arthritis (RA) in one patient, systematic lupus erythematosus (SLE) in another, or neither disorder. The same agent and mechanisms that cause inflammation of the synovial tissues in one patient may cause inflamed kidneys or both disorders in another SLE patient.

Rheumatism may be either inflamed tissues or the result of inflammation, such as synovitis, carditis, or nephritis. When inflammation persists, it may result in chronic rheumatoid disorders.

6

Of all the essential organs, the blood supply is truly our lifeline and first line of defense. It efficiently distributes oxygen, chemicals, hormones, and heat to and from all tissues. The blood supply may determine the primary site of disease activity, such as the kidney or liver, and whether it is localized or widespread. Some tissues are more vulnerable to the inflammatory vascular disorders because they are very highly vascularized (synovium, eye, and kidney). The constriction and restriction of blood supply by inflamed and swollen tissues become life-threatening if they override the automatic control of blood pressure and volume. An adequate venous return of waste products from the tissues and organs is vital to good health.

The life, death, or sickness of every tissue and organ depends on many thousands of closely balanced chemical reactions that interact in a cascading flow or chain reaction. Every cell in the tissue uses the materials supplied by the blood and surrounding cells that were acquired topically or ingested. Also of vital importance and immediate concern in rheumatoid diseases is the inflammatory destruction of the collagen proteins that hold the cells together as functional connective tissues (synovia, blood vessel, and skin).

When a foreign agent enters the synovial joint tissue via the blood stream, the body's defense system, the immune system, will respond. How this highly complex system responds has been a central question of immunology since its beginning. The immune system basically has two components: the cellular and the humoral (or antibody) responses. The major white blood cells involved are lymphocytes (T and B cells), macrophages, and granulocytes.

The body's first line of defense against an invader is to send in an army of white blood cells called neutrophils or granulocytes that flock to the site of invasion, surround the culprit, and release destructive enzymes. This excessive cellular activity results in the release of chemicals and heat that promote reddening, swelling, and pain in the surrounding nerves and tissues. A specific response largely depends on the nature of the offending agent, be it a parasite, virus, bacteria, mycoplasma, or foreign object.

T cells have a surveillance function and immunologic memory. If the memory T cells recognize the agent from a previous infection or vaccination, the body can respond quickly to clear the agent with a coordinated attack from the B cells, which produce specific antibodies or protein molecules that can bind to and coat a foreign molecule (antigen). Antibody-coated antigens are more attractive to the macrophage cells, which can engulf and digest the immune complex (antibody-antigen complex) to remove it from the body. In rheumatoid disease, the offending agent seems to stimulate overkill by turning on uncontrollable and persistent immunologic reactions in different tissues.

Today, there is a growing field of hormonal or cytokine research. This is the study of the patterns of specific protein molecules that T cells release in response to particular signals that occur in an infection or chronic disease, which could provide some insight into the immunologic mechanisms found in arthritis patients. Studies are under way to determine the cytokine patterns found in different tissues of arthritis patients. The results could dramatically increase our understanding of the inflammatory mechanism involved in rheumatoid disease.

Although we cannot readily see inflammation in deep internal tissues (heart, liver, and kidney), the smaller peripheral joints can demonstrate red, hot, swollen, and tender joints. Rheumatism is further distinguished by early morning stiffness, which is not the lack of lubricating oils in the joints, as some have contended. In fact, many joints can accumulate large amounts of fluid that must be drained. This temporary stiffness can become permanent when immobility or lack of exercise fails to keep an adequate blood supply moving throughout the joint's surrounding tendons and muscles. The collagenous joint substance is similar to gelatin proteins that become viscous and stiffens when it cools down while resting. Thus soaking the stiff joints in a warm bath usually restores flexibility. Great relief can also be provided by massaging the muscles to bring more warm blood to the surface, which also increases the essential nourishment of muscles and surrounding tissues. The old maxim holds: use or lose your muscles.

Many patients with rheumatoid arthritis have reported years of fatigue and depression prior to developing any noticeable joint problems and had a hard time convincing their physicians that it was not psychological. Having a realistic idea of what causes symptoms like chronic fatigue, pain, and depression can help patients better

8

control and cope with them. If the early stages of a chronic disease like rheumatism could be recognized before irreversible damage has occurred, therapy could be much more effective. The chronic fatigue syndrome observed in rheumatoid patients may not be a separate disease but like headaches and joint pain is an early warning sign of a body weakened by a persistent battle with the cause of the disease.

Major Medical and Social Problem
Rheumatoid arthritis is the most costly disease afflicting all segments of our population, resulting in an enormous social and economic burden on both the patients and their families. While only one in seven may have some form of arthritis, the other six have to work, play, feed, clothe, and live with them. A major financial consequence of a chronic debilitating and costly disease like arthritis in a majority of our senior citizens has been the serious erosion of our social security system.

Although seldom listed as the cause of death, chronic rheumatoid disease substantially reduces life expectancy as well as forces early retirement on millions. Costly treatments continue to take a large portion of Medicaid and Medicare reserves, contributing to increased private insurance premiums. The trend toward reduced hospital stays after surgery, such as in hip replacements, greatly raises the out-of-pocket expense for rehabilitative nursing care needed during recuperation.

New medicines are extremely expensive, largely because of the enormous cost of drug development, clinical testing and exorbitant profits. When a costly new medicine only provides temporary relief, the desperate patients spend additional billions searching blindly for relief. Many patients have fallen prey to countless dangerous forms of quackery (food fads and remedies) and have developed a very unhealthy skepticism of new approaches and therapy. New untested therapies are frequently listed under quackery, making research and evaluation of their potential benefits more difficult. The effectiveness of tetracycline in rheumatoid arthritis was first reported in 1949 at the 7th International Rheumatology Congress and in the *Journal of Laboratory and Clinical Medicine*. However, the use of tetracycline to treat rheumatoid

9

arthritis has been listed under quackery because it was not adequately tested in double-blind study. At this writing, tetracycline is finally being extensively tested at several clinics. The published results of its benefits support our early findings.

Defining arthritis is extremely complex. However extensivly or narrowly we define arthritis with its hundreds of symptomatic variations we still do not completely describe the numerous associated problems. Many books have been written describing the various forms or types of arthritis in an attempt to help patients understand which type they have and what kind of treatment is available. Unfortunately, it is not that simple, since every patient has a dif-ferent genetic makeup. Not only are there various stages, such as early and late, probable, definite, classic, acute, progressive, and remission, which can vary from day to day, visit to visit, and person to person, but also mixtures and blends with constant diagnostic revisions or updates.

Patients can have rheumatoid arthritis without the arthritis, which means that they have other nonarticular symptoms without any noticeable joint problems. With only fatigue and depression, patients may have a hard time convincing their doctors that it is not psychological. Adults can have Juvenile Rheumatoid Arthritis and children can have adult forms, which may indicate that there are mature and immature immunologic responses to the same agent. Further complicating the problem is that the prescribed medications for one disease have been found to initiate or shift symptoms to another form of arthritis, such as SLE.

To say that the causes and cures of arthritis or the rheumatoid diseases are unknown but soon will be found is a hopeless answer. Researchers have come a lot closer, but closeness does not count for much unless we know what we are close to. If only the researchers and doctors know the questions and answers, the patients, who are in jeopardy, cannot communicate with them. Unless the patients have some idea or understanding of what arthritis is, their input and consideration will continue to be severely limited.

Many doctors would like to slip out the back door when they see rheumatoid disease patients limp into their office. What do doctors tell their failing patients who ask if they should try another clinic? Do they tell patients about the rationale behind the various therapies available and what they will and will not do? After all, patients want their doctor to provide a cure and will do and say almost anything for help. Patients desperately want the medicine to help and hope that they will not be one of the many unfortunate failures. Patients should know that most laboratory tests also measure the activity of several disease mechanisms while helping doctors to evaluate therapeutic effectiveness and the mechanisms of potential causative agents.

When rheumatoid diseases can variably affect one or more tissues and organs and not just the joints, it is understandable why the causes and cures have remained one of medicine's great mysteries. Where do the researchers begin to measure and control all of the contributing factors? How do they evaluate the safety and effectiveness of medications when only the resulting symptoms and not the underlying causes and mechanisms are being measured? The following chapters will explore just how close researchers are to answering "Why Arthritis?"

Chapter II
The Beginning of Arthritis

I n searching for answers concerning arthritis, it is necessary to go back to the beginning. By retracing the steps of previous investigations from the scientific literature, we can verify and establish solid pieces of information on which to build new knowledge, especially those that have withstood the test of time. What we learn depends on our choice and application of new information and ideas. Throughout medical history, major medical advances (such as antiseptics, insulin, and penicillin) have only been accepted after many years of skepticism and inquisition. Long periods of skepticism and doubt are the rule before inclusion in textbooks. Some approved therapies later were shown to be harmful, whereas other therapies, such as tetracycline that were dismissed were later retested and found to be helpful.

Arthritis is one of the oldest diseases. The skeletal remains and fossils of the earliest prehistoric reptiles have degenerative or erosive skeletal changes resembling osteoarthritis in humans. Degenerative skeletons of both large and small prehistoric terrestrial animals suggest that arthritis was not limited to any one species or period or caused by wear and tear or inevitable old age. Whether it was caused by the food they did or did not eat, being warm or cold blooded, or genetic programming, the arthritis was apparently still selective. Not all specimens show degenerative skeletons, indicating a limited susceptibility to at least one agent or condition.

Arthritis in Early Civilization

Arthritis in humans has appeared in one form or another since the earliest recordings of civilization. The Egyptians illustrated the occurrence and treatment of arthritis thousands of years ago and left proof in their carefully preserved mummies.

Hippocrates, the father of medicine, is credited with the original description of arthritis in the fourth century B.C. Using the term *rheums*, which meant flowing or migrating from joint to joint. The Greeks used *rheums* interchangeably with *catarrhos*, which meant flowing down. As we now know, fluid frequently accumulates in the joint, heart, and lung cavities of rheumatoid patients. The brain, which is cushioned in water, was believed to be the source of these humors. Surprisingly, recent literature again emphasizes the brain's control of many immunologic disorders.

Gout

The term gout was derived from *gutta*, Latin for drop. An analogous term was used in 13th century Europe in the "flowing of gouty humur." The term gout was used nonspecifically for many centuries as arthritis is today. The term rheumatism to describe the various joint diseases and other nonmusculoskeletal symptoms was first used in the 17th century. William Heberden (1802) realized how difficult it was to distinguish specific rheumatoid diseases when he wrote:

> *Rheumatism is a common name for many aches and pains which have yet got no peculiar appellation (identity), though owing to very different causes. It is besides often hard to be distinguished from some which have a certain name and class assigned them.*

Gout was a synonym for arthritis until the 17th century, when attacks were thought to arise from gastronomic and sexual excesses. Chemists determined the composition of urinary stones (uric acid crystals) in patients suffering from gout nearly a century after Anton van Leeuwenhoek first used his microscope to detect crystals in gouty tissues.

14

The constant struggle to identify specific types of rheumatism was continued over the past century as doctors keep revising the criteria as to what constitutes rheumatoid arthritis. We are constantly reminded that there are over 100 different forms of arthritis with various combinations of symptoms and few known causes. Questioning what agents and how some cause the characteristic symptoms that seem to wax and wane with increasing severity and complexity has led to the investigation of risk factors and a variety of suspected causes that will be discussed later. Most of what is known about the potential causes of the various symptoms has come in the past 50 years as the result of a major impetus at the beginning of the 20th century to look for the involvement of organs and tissues besides the joints as newer techniques and procedures became available.

Rheumatic Fever
Although rheumatic heart disease was first suggested by Hippocrates, it was not associated with organic heart disease and damaged heart valves until the 19th century as a symptom of acute articular rheumatism. Some years later when tonsillitis was reported to be a common precursor to rheumatic fever, investigators isolated a streptococcal bacteria from a patient's tonsils. Although several bacterial agents were implicated, Homer F. Swift, at the Rockefeller Institute (1928), theorized that rheumatic fever was caused by hypersensitivity (allergy-like responses) to a bacterium. The specific type of beta-hemolytic streptococcus was identified in 1931. This organism is a common cause of sore throats, although not all strep throats result in rheumatic fever. A few years after this great advance in medical history, a young resident physician, Thomas McPherson Brown, went to study with Swift in the hopes of finding the infectious agent causing hypersensitivity in rheumatoid arthritis (1937).

Rheumatoid Arthritis
In 1922, the British Ministry of Health adopted rheumatoid arthritis (RA) as the official designation of the disease first coined by Garrod in 1858; however, the American Rheumatism Association did not accept the name until 1941. The search for a bacterial

cause of RA was in high gear during the 1920s and 1930s and led to the introduction of gold therapy, still used today. In the preantibiotic era, gold salts were used to combat the tuberculosis bacillus, then the suspected cause of RA.

In 1929, sera from 94 percent of RA patients were found to agglutinate or clump suspensions of the streptococcal bacteria isolated from many patients, leading Russel L. Cecil to conclude that RA was the result of streptococcal infection. However, some patients' sera were found to nonspecifically clump other bacteria, even sheep red blood cells coated with normal serum gamma globulin. This early test for the rheumatoid factor that measures the amount of antibody to gamma globulin in some 80 percent of patients with rheumatoid arthritis has been modified and improved over the years. Fifty years later, rheumatologists still do not know what causes 80 percent of patients to produce antibodies against their own antibodies, an obvious immunologic defect. Recent studies in our laboratory indicate a possible mechanism and cause of this rheumatoid factor as well as other autoantibodies produced, which are discussed in another chapter.

Systematic Lupus Erythematosus
The early recognition and classification of other forms of rheumatic disease include systemic lupus erythematosus (SLE), or lupus, a term describing the facial skin rash that resembles a wolf-like mask. The more severe and life-threatening forms of SLE, endocarditis and renal failure, were only recognized in this century. Lupus is considered a classic immune complex disorder because of deposition of gamma globulin in the kidneys. Rheumatoid arthritis, SLE, and progressive systemic sclerosis (PSS) are also classified as collagen vascular or connective tissue disorders because the connective tissue that contains collagen protein is the primary target in these diseases. Lupus is frequently diagnosed with two laboratory tests, the lupus erythematosus cell test and its precursor, the antinuclear antibody activity. Like rheumatoid arthritis, the antinuclear antibodies make lupus another self-destructing autoimmune disorder.

Progressive Systemic Sclerosis
Scleroderma was first observed in the mid 19th century in a young woman with an unusual skin thickening. Over the years, other sys-

tems (renal, heart, lungs, esophagus, and viscera) were recognized as manifestations, which led to the more appropriate designation PSS. The cause of the deposition of collagen in the skin and other tissues remains unknown. The mechanism seems to be the reverse biochemical reaction of that in rheumatoid arthritis: excessive collagen production is found in PSS, whereas in rheumatoid arthritis, the breakdown of collagen by collagenase enzyme from inflammation causes tissue atrophy and destruction. As in most other rheumatoid diseases, some genetic alteration or aberration seems to induce greater susceptibility and predisposition to certain disease mechanisms.

Chapter III
Research Directions

I n searching for answers to the suspected multiple causes and the cures of arthritis, we must first determine the directions we can afford and those that will yield a reachable target and goal. Wild goose chases usually are not very productive unless by sheer luck and the greatest odds you happen to win the lottery, but even those millions will not cure your arthritis. Some still use the shotgun approach, sending investigators out in all directions hoping that someone will find the answers. To determine the best direction and not hit all the dead ends found by other investigators, it is essential to review the course and benchmarks that others have pursued.

Like hunting or fishing, it helps to have some idea of what you are searching for and trying to catch. Do we focus on the primary cause or pursue the contributing risk factors and resulting symptoms? Good hunters rely on the experiences of others as well as their own to help focus on a target.

Risk Factors and Suspected Causes

In 1965, we obtained a large research grant from the Department of Health, Education, and Welfare (HEW), now Health and Human Services (HHS), to investigate a computerized cluster analysis of several thousand parameters that were known or suspected of contributing to or associated with arthritis i.e. RA and SLE. We thought that the computer could tell us which points or parameters were essential for the related disorders. These included the hundreds of both widely and rarely used diagnostic tests as well as the many forms of exposures at home, work, and play, from alcohol and asbestos to an extensive psychosocial analysis. Because some infectious agents were highly suspect, serologic blood tests were also included to determine possible exposure.

From the hundred patients extensively measured, the computer reemphasized that no two were identical and at least 100 symptomatic parameters could be found in a majority of the RA patients. Whatever the causes, this suggested that we could not identify a simple winning combination or cluster in all patients. Primarily because of our interest in the potential role of infectious agents, especially mycoplasmas, the serologic tests, as previously reported, were positive in many but not all. The current tissue and genetic typing and other more sensitive high-tech tests were not available at that time. The results of these studies unfortunately were reported but never published and were later used by the National Arthritis Advisory Board in 1976 when they established a master data collection plan for arthritis research.

Although there may be other unknown risk factors, they are apparently very rare in common forms of arthritis. Just as excessive sunlight can worsen some forms of arthritis, excessive darkness with the lack of vitamin D (ultraviolet irradiated calciferol) may retard bone metabolism. Except for inactivity, poor dietary habits are probably the greatest risk factor and, like the hormonal release from physical or mental stress, can precipitate chronic and acute arthritis. This is found especially in cases of food and other allergies, which can exacerbate preexisting hypersensitivity reactions of RA. Allergies can also limit tolerance to medications. The failure to exercise or massage the muscles will not provide the vital stimulation of blood vessels and their life-supporting circulation. These and other factors will be discussed later in therapy evaluation.

It is easy to keep saying that we do not know the causes of arthritis and continue promising that we will succeed with more research support. This has been the theme and hallmark of most arthritis research plans for the past 25 years. Unless the suspected

20

and potential causes are targeted, investigated, and either ruled in or out, we will still be searching the haystacks and not know what the cause of rheumatic disorders looks like.

Because of the great importance of finding the cause, I once naively suggested to the National Institutes of Health (NIH) that all investigators should focus their research efforts on whatever they considered to be the most probable cause, whether metabolic, hormonal, genetic, viral, bacterial, or mycoplasmal. Perhaps this way we could narrow the field to the major suspects. This suggestion actually was not too far off, since most investigators are limited in their experience and field of research. The major barrier to finding the cause lies in the experts' inability to pursue a new direction outside their discipline, which requires a major team effort. Besides, researchers like to pursue positive projects with no dead ends that will yield publications and thus assure continued grant renewals. We now know that viral and mycoplasmal research are not compatible and must be studied separately. Although there is a good possibility of multiple infections, a combination cannot be dismissed and will be discussed later as the potential role and mechanisms of infectious agents.

After determining what to search for, the next problem is where to search. The choices are the human patient, animal models, and tissue cultures. Looking for the causative agent in test tubes under carefully controlled conditions may be the most scientifically controlled research but is the least significant and relevant to the complex human host. Testing for a potential infectious cause in tissue cell or organ cultures could reveal certain biological reactions and mechanisms that are not comparable in humans. In some infectious diseases, the experimental animal model has been most helpful in proving the microbial cause, which is often referred to as fulfilling Koch's postulates.

Fortunately, all animals do not respond to human diseases, and humans do not catch all animal diseases. A good example was the recent discovery of Lyme disease or Lyme arthritis, which is caused by a microbial spirochete transmitted in bites from ticks that are carried by deer, mice, and other furry animals that apparently do not develop Lyme arthritis. Although investigators have found that the animal strains of mycoplasmas can cause arthritis in certain animals, they have not been found to be reactive in humans. The animal models provide researchers with promising directions regarding where, when, and how to look for a cause and even test treatment. The use of animal models of arthritis will be discussed in a subsequent chapter. The cause of rheumatic disease in elephants and the great apes, the closest human model, was investigated. Having found mycoplasmas to cause arthritis in animals, veterinarians have been able to successfully control animal arthritis with antibiotic (tetracycline) therapy.

Because research on humans is far more complex and costly, making it more difficult to search for causes and cures, it has had to take a back seat to the more scientific animal models. Most of the research on patients has focused on measuring and testing symptoms that are the result of disease mechanisms and not the cause. Most of the studies have centered around the arthritic joints, synovial joint fluid, and tissues, together with a detailed analysis of the venous blood supply leaving the inflamed tissues. Where and what parts of the body do you search for the causative agent, especially in a disease that can be localized to one joint or systemically dispersed to many tissues and organs? In one study, we found the suspected mycoplasma localized in one knee joint that had not yet spread to the other knee or peripheral blood. In other patients, we have isolated mycoplasmas from the chest fluid, ovaries, and other tissues. Should you or could you investigate every tissue and joint or just those showing inflammation? The restrictions on investigating fetal tissue, where the earliest cause and onset of RA may occur, greatly hamper research.

Susceptibility to arthritis has even been linked to the brain's regulation of inflammation. Work at NIH showed that differences in the body's response to stress play a major role in the susceptibility and resistance to the development of arthritis, at least in two strains of rats. The researchers reported that the defect is in the brain's hypothalamus and its ability to produce a hormone critical in regulating the response to (not the cause of) inflammation. This finding is consistent with the concept that the brain has a controlling effect on the development of arthritis. Along these lines, it is interesting to note that there have been reports of a much higher incidence of rheumatoid disorders in mental hospital patients.

Should senility or dementia brain disorders, even Alzheimer's and multiple sclerosis, be included in rheumatoid research? Is there a rheumatoid disorder of the brain associated with neurovascular disorders?

Prior to 1949, when corticosteroids were introduced, many researchers were looking at personality types as the basis of arthritis. Even today, the hard-driving, competitive, hostility trait may be the cause of high blood pressure with vascular (blood vessel) damage, resulting in rheumatoid as well as coronary and cerebral diseases. We did not need an expert or a double blind controlled study to show us that laughter is good medicine, as *Reader's Digest* has so often reported. Today, we know that love can cure and that hate is suicidal.

Apparently, we have good hormones and not so good hormones that can turn our systems on or off with the control or cause of inflammation. If the rheumatoid disease mechanisms are lying dormant, the wrong or too much hormone stimulant could fan the flames, causing the disease to erupt like a volcano. If the disease is active and boiling, the release of corticosteroids or an anti-inflammatory hormone could quickly reduce the heat but not the fire. An extensive psychosocial evaluation of RA patients has found that rheumatoid disease can markedly change a patient's personality. Contrary to belief, the disease also was shown to be reversible with therapeutic remission.

Is old age a cause or a risk factor? The musculoskeletal symptoms of aches and fatigue comprise the most common conditions affecting the elderly. Surveys of this problem indicate that arthritis is the most common medical complaint among the elderly. Unlike younger people, elderly patients begin to express a wide range of disorders that seemingly are outside the range of rheumatic diseases. These include malignancies and endocrine, metabolic, neurologic, and vascular disorders. Arthritis or degenerative joint disease actually may be only one of the many manifestations of the chronic and progressive rheumatoid diseases.

Thus to sort out a primary cause from the many contributing risk factors, investigators must look at the earliest onset of rheumatoid diseases to find out what started first—the arthritis or the nonarticular symptoms. Should research focus on the infant, the young female, or the elderly? In an effort to find and identify an infectious cause of rheumatoid diseases, it has been suggested that patients should be studied at the earliest onset of symptoms. Although promising, this research direction could be difficult to pursue because it would have to introduce young children as research subjects and not just the elderly, since their arthritis may have started many years ago with some childhood disease or at birth.

Contrary to the theory that overweight equals wear and tear, underweight patients were recently reported to have a significantly higher risk of severe outcome. Perhaps the arthritis was of thyroid origin or due to gastromalabsorption, resulting in a nutritional deficiency of the joint tissues and muscles. The fact that weak muscles can leave the joints in a very precarious and compromised position should be of great concern for the elderly. If muscle atrophy or wasting leads to traumatic arthritis and broken bones, then perhaps we should be looking for its causes, which might also promote the related loss of calcium in osteoporosis.

Many factors contributing to general poor health can also contribute to the aches and fatigue of rheumatoid disorders. Whether gastrointestinal problems were caused by the patients' medications and contributed to the onset and proliferation of their disease presents another formidable problem for both patients and doctors. Because of the unpredictable course of rheumatoid disease, except for being cyclic, progressive, and down hill, the probable cause and risk factors are difficult to relate to the disease onset. This raises an important question of whether to search for the cause in the very young or the more afflicted elderly. A lot of rheumatoid patients are needed to evaluate therapy. This usually includes nonchild-bearing elderly females in the earliest stages without any complications or associative symptoms. Unfortunately, clinical drug trials require only those patients with classic symptoms, especially in multiple joints, in order to detect significant therapeutic changes. The cause may be some triggering or inactive agent that was present years ago, as some have suggested. The one active agent is now gone or deeply buried, perhaps in a cyst, and no longer isolated and detected.

Geneticists are trying to predict whether people will develop a certain type of arthritis based on their tissues' susceptibility or predisposition to the unknown cause. The genetic contribution or defect will be discussed in a subsequent chapter on causes. For the present time, the role of genetics as an inevitable noncontrollable factor determines who is more susceptible to an infectious agent or which one of the identical twins will develop rheumatoid arthritis or SLE. That one twin was delivered first or birth weights of twins are different provides a whole series of extrinsic conditions in their ensuing lives that may shift the reactions to a favorable or un-favorable outcome. A specific tissue type seems to be only one of many predisposing or contributing factors and not a cause by itself. Thus putting all our eggs in the genetic research basket does not seem to provide a fertile area in which to find the cause or cure. Having to screen thousands of donors to find a perfect bone marrow match further indicates the magnitude of dissimilarity among the patients at risk.

What Decides the Research Direction

The statistical results of the 1950 U.S. Population Health survey indicated that young, nonwhite females with low incomes in rural areas would have the highest incidence of arthritis. Some 40 years later, this prognosis is still partially true, especially if you consider certain forms of arthritis, such as RA and SLE. The suburban sprawl, with the introduction of electricity, water, sewers, the telephone, television, and the automobiles has greatly reduced the rural geographic boundaries, replacing them with inner cities and new and unknown risk factors.

The greater geographical incidence of some forms of arthritis in other parts of the world is usually attributable to markedly different social customs and mores. Higher rates of diseases, such as tuberculosis, leprosy, and malaria, attributable to malnutrition, poor sanitation, and other adverse living conditions surprisingly limit rather than enhance the incidence of rheumatic diseases. Bacteria, viruses, tuberculosis, leprosy, and other known infectious agents that cause infections or septic arthritis, although similar, are not the same chronic and persistent mechanisms that cause rheumatic diseases. Thus the search for the unknown cause would be simplified by investigating patients living in areas having fewer infectious diseases and complicating problems.

Usually the advisory and peer-review councils, funding

agencies, foundations, and institutions have the final say in what research direction is worthy of support. The International League Against Rheumatism (ILAR), comprised of national rheumatology organizations in countries around the world, meets every four years to compare clinical and basic research findings, often in conjunction with the World Health Organization (WHO). ILAR and WHO do not provide arthritis research funds per se, but their worldwide influence can focus attention and interest on a particular therapy and research direction. Although similarities and differences are found, no race or genetic type is exempt from rheumatic disease, as the origin and cause remain unknown. Some may claim that the United States has the best medical care in the world. However, it also has some of the most crippling forms of arthritis and the most costly, with nothing much more to show for it, not even greater longevity.

Several research reports presented to ILAR by our research group over the past 40 years (1949-1989) will be discussed in other chapters, as well as a discussion of the costs and benefits of research and therapy. Except for the new and exotic forms of testing and therapy, the search for possible causes and risk factors has not been very active or productive. The newer forms of therapy, have not provided unified directions or results, while aspirin remains the drug of first choice. However, one group of therapeutic agents, the multiple-action tetracyclines, will be discussed later with therapies that point toward a very probable cure and cause.

Therapeutic successes and failures have had an important role in determining research direction. The discovery of pleuro-pneumonia-like organisms (PPLO), now known as mycoplasmas, in humans by Louis Dienes in 1932 was soon followed by their isolation from arthritic mice by Albert Sabin (of polio fame) in 1938 at the Rockefeller Institute. Taking this new direction a step further, Thomas McPherson Brown, also at the Rockefeller Institute and searching for an infectious cause of rheumatic diseases, reported in 1938 the isolation of mycoplasmas from a patient's rheumatic tissues. Although there is little doubt about mycoplasmas causing arthritis in mice, rats, pigs, and many other animals, they remain only a suspect in human rheumatoid diseases. Sabin found that not only did gold salts inhibit mycoplasmal growth but more importantly reduced inflammatory arthritis in mycoplasma-infected mice

26

and rats. The gold therapy frequently used today was introduced in the 1920s when tuberculosis was the suspected cause of rheumatoid disease.

The belief that mycoplasmas were the cause and gold salts were the cure for rheumatoid disease was abandoned by World War II, especially since mycoplasmas could not be readily isolated from all the rheumatoid patients. Furthermore, gold therapy was quite toxic and not effective in all rheumatoid patients. Again, the research direction shifted to other areas, such as the beneficial effects of sulfur compounds and especially the miraculous corticosteroids, indicating some hormonal or metabolic deficiency. This metabolic direction was emphasized and supported with the establishment of the new Arthritis and Metabolic Institute at NIH. For several years, NIH promoted corticosteroid therapy as the most promising research direction.

Fortunately, a few researchers were not deterred by this shift in direction. In 1949, Dienes reported to the 7th International Rheumatology Congress the isolation of mycoplasmas from the genitourinary tracts of arthritic males. In discussing the significance of this observation, Brown reported his successful treatment of 17 rheumatoid patients with the new tetracycline antibiotic (Aureomycin), which had recently been found, like gold salts (not penicillin), to inhibit mycoplasmal growth. At the same international Congress, reports on the miraculous treatment of rheumatoid patients with cortisone attracted most of the attention and publicity while detracting from the other research directions reported by Dienes and Brown. The beneficial response to cortisone led to the belief that a hormonal deficiency or abnormality was the causative mechanism, as shown by the greater incidence in females. After several years of overdosage, rheumatologists finally realized cortisone's lethal dangers and that it was only suppressing symptoms and not the causative agent or disease.

Basic and Clinical Research
It soon became apparent that two divergent research directions were developing. Basic research projects directed toward a potential microbial cause were separate from clinical studies of therapeutic effectiveness. Consequently, most research efforts to find the causes

and solve the rheumatoid problem have either been directed toward the isolation and identification of a probable microbial cause or clinical studies of symptoms and associative symptomatic therapy, including anti-inflammatory and immunosuppressive drugs. The cause and effect were kept separate in humans. Alhough an infectious agent was highly suspect, antimicrobial therapy was not promoted.

In 1972 a committee sponsored by the Arthritis Foundation summarized the previous 25 years of research, stating that "it was unlikely that a genuinely effective treatment for either the prevention or cure of the disease would be developed until the causes were clearly understood". Based on past experience and available information, our research team had reported 20 years before (1951) on a study of the antigen-antibody mechanism in rheumatic diseases in the *American Journal Medical Science*. Forty years later, we reported on the role and mechanism of mycoplasma immune complexes as the most probable cause of rheumatic diseases. Although other microbial agents can also form immune complexes, they have not been associated with rheumatoid diseases.

In support of research directed toward the infectious agent hypothesis, we reported at a national infectious disease meeting in 1964 finding positive serology (blood test) for mycoplasmal antibodies in most of the rheumatoid patients. Within limitations of the test at that time, such findings would suggest that the patients were or had been infected with one or more of the mycoplasmal strains tested. Further, the results showing that the females were infected four times more frequently than males certainly supported the greater (4:1) incidence of rheumatoid arthritis in females.

As many more microbiologists became interested in the very unusual properties of mycoplasma, the increased efforts to isolate mycoplasmas from inflamed tissues and not just the throat and genitourinary tract were fraught with more negative than positive results. For several years, investigators had tried to identify the atypical virus that caused pneumonia. Unlike most viruses, the so-called Viral Eaton agent, like mycoplasmas, was inhibited by tetracyclines. In 1962, primarily because of the agent's tetracycline sensitivity, investigators at NIH were able to isolate and identify the atypical viral agent as a mycoplasma. Because it caused atypical pneumonia in humans, it was named *Mycoplasma pneumoniae.*

This observation aroused the interest of many investigators who had given up and considered mycoplasmas, at least the human strains, as nonpathogenic or nondisease-causing agents. This conclusion was reasonable because several years earlier our research group had discovered mycoplasmas growing unknowingly in tissue cell cultures without killing the tissue cells. These were the same tissue cell cultures used by virologists to culture viruses and prepare viral vaccines, such as those used for polio and measles.

Unfortunately, the nonkilling mycoplasma contamination of tissue cell cultures still remains a foremost problem for the virologist and mycoplasmologist. More importantly, it demonstrates that mycoplasmas can and do live symbiotically, at least with some test tube tissues, as a noninfectious pathogen. This observation is comparable to the frequent isolation of mycopalasmas from the throats and genital tracts of asymptomatic or healthy people.

Who Decides the Research Direction?
Faced with the unknown genesis of the infectious causes of many chronic and degenerative diseases, NIH brought together the heads of medical departments and the scientific communities at four regional meetings in 1965. The objective was to solicit and discuss their views on the role of infectious agents and immunologic reactions together with suggested areas and methods for research.

The enthusiasm manifested at these meetings amply justified the suspicion that a significant amount of information was available to warrant participation of the scientific community leaders in a broad frontal attack on the infectious and immunologic genesis of chronic and degenerative diseases, including the rheumatoid diseases. The fact that many of the participants had not previously given serious thought to this subject and hence had limited experience, was a contributing factor in limiting the discussion of proposed direction and action.

Many participants expressed the opinion that solid evidence or anecdotal inferences existed for a microbial cause of some of these diseases. A number of participants stated that evidence of the role of an infectious agent in rheumatoid arthritis was clear but unknown. Our representative, Brown, expressed the view that solving such problems as rheumatoid arthritis would be more likely if one pursued a potential infectious cause and mechanism rather than trying to arrive at a solution based only on symptoms or the results of the disease. A few participants believed that animal model systems represented exact counterparts of human diseases. Others believed that even though there were no absolute counterparts, a study of the broad biological mechanisms in animals should be given high priority. A study of the role of animal model systems in future research was projected in these explorative conferences. The contribution of animals in rheumatoid disease research will be reviewed in a subsequent chapter.

Many of the participants at these conferences, sponsored by the National Institute of Allergy and Infectious Diseases (NIAID), serve on the various research review councils that decide the priority and funding of research grant applications for specific projects. Based on their knowledge and experience in a particular area, they must decide on the merits and feasibility of the proposed research direction. Unfortunately, the peer reviewers are not always knowledgeable of the many recent and as yet unpublished basic and clinical observations. Thus support for research in the known or familiar areas is given preference over a new and unknown direction as a less secure investment.

With the establishment and rapid development of NIH in the 1950s and 1960s, supported by the ever-increasing federal funds, the production of biological and medical research findings was explosive. Perhaps the greatest fallout has been the vast separation of the interdisciplinary specialties, particularly between basic researchers and applied clinicians. This directional problem was particularly noted at the 1965 NIH conferences. It was acknowledged that the multidisciplinary nature of the chronic disease research would make communications difficult but vital.

The family doctor and basic research groups now have great barriers in exchanging new information and problems understanding each other. The rapid increase in the number of specialty medical journals illustrates the expanding difficulties of under-standing and communicating on a common wave-length. Even in 1964, our attempt to obtain NIH grant support for a combined basic and applied clinical research project had to take a long circuitous route

30

through both the basic and clinical review councils, resulting in a lengthy final decision as to which institute could, should, or would fund it. When it was finally approved, we had already obtained private support elsewhere and could not accept the duplicating NIH award. Grant applications require detailed blue-prints of the proposed research project with significant evidence and justification for success. In order to develop and provide details of a new research direction with substantial justification and feasibility, prior studies, often extensive, are required. Such studies require the need for the essential funding of early and high-risk preliminary studies. Such critical funding is often provided by universities' general funds, private nonprofit organizations, and patients.

Originally, the federal grants from NIH were for short-term support of 1 to 3 years. When the research is directed toward long-term chronic diseases, the early termination of grants or renewal failure forces investigators to seek private support in order to salvage the vital and as yet unpublished information. In times when research funds are greatly limited and more highly competitive, it is instinctive and essential that investigators limit the details of their projects, even though the information is marked confidential so that new ideas and directions are not provided to their competitors, the peer reviewers.

The competition for support in chronic disease research, especially rheumatoid diseases, pits research for killers versus that for cripplers and nonkillers. A good example is the astronomical support given to AIDS research without a unified direction, which was the prestigious position formerly occupied by cancer and heart disease whose cause and cure remain unknown. That arthritis is the nation's number one crippler and one of the most costly major socioeconomic problems affecting untold millions of people still does not warrant a fair share of the available public research funds. Obviously, the millions and now billions spent each year on the killer diseases without a meaningful research direction toward their cause and cure still have not bought a solution.

Private funding from charitable foundations for chronic disease research is limited and usually restricted to specific diseases or general health care. Like the Arthritis Foundation, many of these disease-related foundations depend on charitable contributions from long-suffering patients and their families and friends. How much of their funds are directed toward basic or clinical research is highly variable. For example, in 1983, the Arthritis Foundation's priorities were public information, professional education, public education, patient services, professional training, and lastly research. With no funds designated for research, the AF terminated our research support that year.

The force and effectiveness of these national health organizations are further splintered into many special interest disease groups (such as osteoarthritis, lupus, juvenile, muscle, and kidney), which want support directed toward their particular anatomical symptoms and not the whole patient. Hundreds of non-profit medical groups continue to proliferate in the face of minimal advances while spending millions of dollars each year with no solutions or even a solid direction toward their problem, only more costly band aid therapy. Of course finding a solution or cure for their particular disease could put them out of business.

Chapter IV
Why Do Animals Have Arthritis?

After many years of neglected communications, veterinarians and medical professionals have joined forces, much to their patients' benefits. The resulting field of comparative medicine continues to be one of the most rewarding areas in opening new doors and finding answers. Discovering the cause of arthritis in animals should certainly help in finding the cause in humans. Although there are great physiological and metabolic differences between most animals and humans, the accepted scientific proof of the cause of a human disease has been its reproduction in animals. Ironically, this cardinal rule put forth by Robert Koch, known as Koch's postulate, was initiated in the late 19th century when Louis Pasteur and other microbiologists were isolating and identifying the microbial causes of smallpox, chickenpox, rabies, and other acute infectious diseases.

More recently, there has been increased concern, especially in zoological parks, about humans sharing diseases, such as tuberculosis, with animals. As a result, nonhuman primates are observed behind glass walls in many zoos to prevent disease transmission. Arthritis in domestic animals, unlike the human varieties, is usually contagious, with rapid debilitation and often fatal outcome, requiring euthanasia if not treated early. With no one to feed them, arthritic animals are too crippled to get to their food. Arthritic

33

elephants can never lie down, knowing their crippled hind legs will not lift them back up. Without all of their assisting devices, humans might well suffer the same fate as animals.

One of the earliest reports on a cause of animal arthritis was made by scientists at the Pasteur Institute in 1898 who had isolated a new microbe, bovis pleuropneumonia, the causative agent of a fatal pneumonia and arthritis in cattle. These viral-like microbes were highly transmissible and threatened the total loss of cattle throughout the world. This particular strain of pleuropneumonia-like organisms (PPLO), now known as Mycoplasma mycoides, is still forbidden entry into the United States. In the ensuing four decades, veterinarians and microbiologists isolated similar types of mycoplasmas from goats, sheep, chickens, turkeys, pigs, dogs, cats, rats, and mice. Many of these strains were found to cause a variety of arthritic, respiratory, reproductive, and neurologic diseases in different animal species.

PPLOs, now called mycoplasmas, are probably the most prevalent cause of arthritis in animals. Perhaps if it was not for animals' vital agriculture value and the devastating epidemic problems that still potentially exist, concerted efforts to find and eliminate the cause would not have been made. Prior to antibiotics, mycoplasma vaccines were prepared and used with limited success. Outbreaks of infections usually required the destruction of herds and flocks. Unlike bacteria and viruses, mycoplasmas, especially the human strains, have a chronic pathologic mechanism that is not readily controlled by vaccines.

Apparently, arthritis is not limited to domestic animals. In 1929, Herbert Fox reported his observations on the skeletal remains of many wild animal species. He reported finding the highest incidence of arthritic changes in gorillas, which are the closest primate to humans. The skeletal remains of a dozen mountain gorillas sent to the Smithsonian Institution by the late Dian Fossey revealed evidence of arthritis in gorillas. It is not known whether the natives transmitted a causative agent to the gorillas, although the arthritic gorillas surely would have been easier prey for human poachers.

Although zoos do not like to put their crippled and sick animals on display, they have to rely on public support and recent medical advances to keep their exotic specimens healthy and active.

The irony is that some experimental drugs are often first tested on human patients before veterinarians used them to treat their precious and endangered zoological specimens.

Going Ape With Arthritis

The warm spring sun was shining down through the skylight on a black hairy creature curled up in the corner of its spacious zoo cage. My curiosity was aroused partially because the sign on the cage read a Lowland Gorilla, suggesting a massive animal. My thoughts about whether it was sleeping or sick were short lived, when a zoo attendant entered the cage with a tray full of assorted fruits and vegetables. With some gentle coaxing and holding one arm, the attendant helped a young crippled gorilla walk around the cage to exercise its legs. Quite obviously, touching its left foot to the floor was extremely painful, at least it hurt me to watch him try. I knew from many years in arthritis research that a little exercise was essential. Seeing this dwarfed and severely crippled young gorilla made me wonder why the three other gorillas in neighboring cages were not afflicted. What made it so sad and pathetic was that unlike a child, the gorilla could not tell us where and how much it hurt. What hurt the most was learning that it faced euthanasia, as all 26 of the available arthritis drugs had provided very little relief.

In 1969, 40 years after Fox reported observing the high incidence of arthritis in gorilla skeletons, our arthritis research team at George Washington University reported the diagnosis and successful treatment of a gorilla with severe rheumatoid arthritis at the National Zoo in Washington, D.C. Of particular interest was that the 5-year-old male gorilla, Tomoka, was the fourth gorilla to be born in captivity. Furthermore, his younger brother and sister, who were also born at the National Zoo, were sent to other zoos where they developed arthritis. Neither of their parents had a history of arthritis. However, a specific strain of human-related mycoplasmas isolated from Tomoka's throat was also found by serologic blood tests to have infected his brother and sister. Serum from several other gorillas, orangutans, and chimpanzees in the zoo tested negative for these mycoplasmal antibodies. Whether this mycoplasma, also found in humans, was the causal agent or a very unusual coincidence remains to be proven.

35

Bimonthly intravenous tetracycline therapy proved successful in bringing Tomoka's rheumatoid arthritis into remission. This I.V. antibiotic therapy, which was originally developed and successfully tested in human rheumatoid arthritis patients by Brown, was subsequently used successfully by veterinarians in several other zoos. Although still unproven, we believe that tetracycline therapy was successful in controlling the disease by inhibiting mycoplasma growth and thus eliminating the causal infectious agent.

Three years earlier, in 1966, at an NIH conference on the relationship of mycoplasma to rheumatoid arthritis and related diseases, a rheumatologist asked whether apes got any of these diseases. He suggested that we would be well ahead of the game if a primate model could be found. At that time, the mycoplasmal cause of arthritis in many domestic animal species was well known. Thus in 1969 it should have come as no surprise when we diagnosed and successfully treated the severe rheumatoid arthritis in the gorilla Tomoka, who was infected with a related human strain of mycoplasma. The successful treatment with tetracycline therapy every 2 weeks was based primarily on the most effective and safest therapeutic regimen we had developed for human RA patients over the past 20 years. Tomoka has been a beautiful healthy specimen for over 20 years and has often been featured in cover stories of newspapers and magazines around the world. Perhaps Tomoka will be recognized in medical history as providing the most promising research direction to the cause and cure of rheumatoid disorders. In addition, a young female gorilla (Snickers) at the Philadelphia Zoo who was diagnosed with probable lupus was found to be infected with a human strain of mycoplasmas and was also successfully treated with intermittent intravenous tetracycline. Many other arthritic gorillas in zoos around the world have benefit from this applied clinical research.

Blood specimens from hundreds of great apes (gorillas, orangutans, and chimpanzees) and their human keepers in zoos around the world were tested for mycoplasma infection in our search for a correlation with their arthritic symptoms. Although we could not get blood specimens from the noncaptive apes in Africa, this study compared arthritic symptoms in both captive and noncaptive great apes through communications with scientists observ-

36

ing them in the jungles of Africa and Borneo. According to reports from Dian Fossey, there was a relatively higher incidence of arthritis in the gorillas than the orangutans or chimpanzees. This agreed with our finding a much higher incidence of arthritis in the captive gorillas and also confirms the 1929 report by Fox.

In 1991, after years of delay, NIH finally began working with several medical centers to develop a protocol for an extensive controlled clinical trial of tetracycline in human rheumatoid arthritis patients. The same year, a cover story in the Washington Post again featured the gorilla Tomoka (See p 38).

Because of the biological closeness of gorillas to humans, Tomoka was probably one of the first arthritic animal models whose life was saved by prior human clinical research. As some experts have claimed, the key was not learning to cope with an incurable disease, as Tomoka was unable to change his lifestyle or attend special group therapy courses.

In an effort to confirm our hypothesis, investigators at NIH and a Texas primate center injected a large dose of mycoplasmas from a rheumatoid arthritis patient into a gorilla's knee, producing localized inflammatory arthritis. Unfortunately, such a septic or infectious form of arthritis neither confirms nor proves that myco-plasmas are the cause of the more chronic and systemic rheumatoid arthritis in humans, as the injection of almost any bacteria or foreign material (even charcoal) into a knee joint can produce inflammatory arthritis.

Although mycoplasmas are now accepted as a primary cause of arthritis in gorillas, definitive evidence for the mycoplasma con-nection in human rheumatoid arthritis has proven more elusive, prompting many leading rheumatologists to simply dismiss our theory as unproven. Some rheumatologists still believe that the mycoplasma cause and tetracycline therapy for RA were laid to rest years ago (1971). In fact, tetracycline has not been thoroughly tested until recently.

Other Experimental Animal models
Mice and rats are the two laboratory models of experimental arthritis that have been extensively studied. The injection of killed bacteria, collagen protein, or inert particles into the knee joint

Tomoka

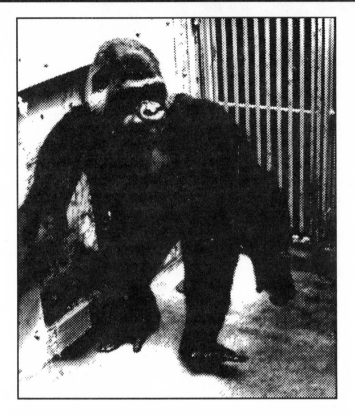

Tomoka, a 29-year-old gorilla in the Washington Zoo, was crippled 25 years ago by a form of arthritis that was striking dozens of large zoo and circus animals, especially great apes and elephants. He was saved by a tetracycline treatment devised by the late rheumatologist, Thomas McPherson Brown. Since then, antibotics have been used routinely to treat arthritis in large animals. Now there is renewed interest in their possible usefulness as a treatment for arthritis in people.

Sandy Rovnar
Washington Post Health
January 15, 1991

causes localized and transient inflammatory arthritis. The injection of a specific strain of mycoplasma isolated from an arthritic rat into a rabbit's knee produces a localized but more chronic form of arthritis. Depending upon the route of entry (respiratory, urogenital, or blood), the injection of viable strains of mycoplasma into mice would result in either pneumonia or arthritis. Some injected mouse strains of mycoplasma produced an uncontrollable rolling motion in mice, fueling speculation for the possible existence of human strains of mycoplasma that may contribute to neurologic disorders in humans, such as Alzheimer's, multiple sclerosis, or encephalitis.

As many pet owners know, cats and dogs often become crippled with arthritis, especially old dogs. These animals have been found to be infected with their own unique feline and canine strains of mycoplasmas. Knowing this, we have encouraged veterinarians and dog owners to try tetracycline therapy. Although not a controlled double-blind study, some of them reported marked improvement and even remission. Some investigators who noted that a high percentage of pet owners had rheumatoid arthritis raised the question whether the pets may have contributed to the cause of human arthritis. Believing that the animal strains of mycoplasmas were species specific and not known to infect humans, we ran extensive blood tests on dog owners and their dogs, especially those with arthritis. As suspected, the dogs were serologically positive for only the canine strains of mycoplasmas, and the owners were only positive for the human strains of mycoplasmas.

In a similar study, we tested the animal caretakers in several zoos, especially the elephant handlers, for antibodies to both the human and elephant mycoplasma strains. Only in one handler, who was asymptomatic, were we able to detect positive antibodies to an elephant mycoplasma. Not finding any significant cross-infectiousness between human and animal mycoplasmas helped to reassure the zoo staff that their arthritis did not come from their animals and vice versa. These observations also showed that the infectious cause of RA was not readily transmitted to family members. We did find that two gorillas who tested negative for mycoplasma antibodies and the rheumatoid factor developed severe arthritis when shipped to another zoo. The arthritic gorillas then tested positive for both mycoplasma antibodies and the rheumatoid factor. Both gorillas responded favorably to intravenous tetracycline therapy and are good examples of shipping fever, frequently found in livestock undergoing the stress of transportation.

When investigators at NIH injected a strain of mycoplasma isolated from arthritic pigs into normal pigs, a chronic form of inflammatory arthritis was produced that persisted even though the mycoplasma could no longer be isolated. Like our previous findings in rheumatoid patients, the pigs' blood and joint fluid tests remained positive for the mycoplasma antibodies. Even though mycoplasmas could no longer be isolated from this experimental swine model after the arthritis surfaced, NIH and peer rheumatologists have insisted that we must identify mycoplasmas in arthritis patients before they would approve and support a double-blind controlled tetracycline trial.

Standards have changed since gold therapy was first administered, when many believed that tuberculosis was the cause of arthritis. Contrary to the experts' previous recommendations, NIH is now supporting the costly clinical trials of oral and intravenous tetracycline therapy and the potential role of mycoplasmas and other infectious etiologies in rheumatoid arthritis.

Unfortunately, very little of the information obtained from the arthritic animal models has been applied to humans, except perhaps for testing anti-inflammatory drugs. This could be one of the greatest failures in medical history. Knowing that mycoplasmas cause arthritis and other disorders in many animal species and are inhibited by the tetracycline antibiotics, especially by intravenous administration, it was never adequately tested in humans. Tragically, even without such studies, the Arthritis Foundation for many years reported in their brochure that "antibiotics do not help rheumatoid arthritis". Antibiotics trials were further discouraged when the Arthritis Foundation listed the untested tetracycline treatment in their articles about quackery and unproven remedies. Many microbiologists still insist that any infectious cause of rheumatoid arthritis in humans should also produce the disease in an animal model. So why not apply the animal model knowledge in reverse?

Animal models have played important roles in searching for

the cause and cure of rheumatoid disorders. In 1989, investigators at NIH reported that the susceptibility to arthritis was linked to the brain's regulation of inflammation. Two species of rats showed different stress-related responses to their hormonal control of adrenocorticotrophin hormone (ACTH) and cortisone blocking their immune responses and thus the amount of inflammation. Cortisone, which is normally released in response to physical and mental stress, suppresses the immune response through its effects on the level of interleukin and cytokine hormones, the mediators of inflammation and cell proliferation. The role of stress may be an important factor in the high incidence of rheumatoid factor positive patients that are found in mental hospitals. Physical and mental stress have been well documented as an associated factor in the onset of rheumatoid disorders. In the early 1930s, when mycoplasmas were first found to cause arthritis in rats, investigators also found that additional physical stress, such as immersion in ice water, contributed to a much higher incidence of arthritis in rats.

Another NIH news release in 1990 reported that a group of researchers using genetic engineering techniques produced a rat model that spontaneously developed a group of arthritic diseases called spondyloarthropathies (spinal arthritis). Fertilized eggs of rats were injected with human DNA containing the genetic marker HLA-B27, a cell surface antigen that is believed to predispose individuals to arthritic disease. The researchers were able to produce an animal model that strikingly mimics nearly all manifestations of the human spinal disease. Because not all patients with these diseases carry this genetic marker in their tissues, these studies may merely confirm the greater predisposition or susceptibility to the suspected primary infectious cause. To determine the role of an infectious agent in the development of this disease in transgenic animal models, studies should include a completely germ-free environment.

Researchers previously had bred specific strains of animals, dogs, and mice that would spontaneously develop arthritis, indicating an inherited genetic cause. However, the validity of these genetic models was challenged when viruses or other infectious agents were found to be carried and transmissible in these animals. Although there are familial or genetic components in rheumatoid disease, there is no proof or evidence that it was ever inherited.

Arthritis in the Beasts of Burden:
Working with veterinarians around the world, we serologically tested blood for antibodies against mycoplasmas and cultured oral and genital tracts for viable mycoplasmas in over 100 circus and zoo elephants. Another 48 elephants from a private farm in Florida, including many juveniles flown in from Africa, were also tested. Just as people feel better when they are doing something enjoyable, so do circus elephants. On cold mornings, some elephants limp, while others are too stiff and sore to move. When it warms up and the band starts playing, the elephants all walk briskly into the center ring, and no one notices which elephants have rheumatoid disorders. A good example was the arthritic elephant Mary who tapped the spring board with her front leg and sent her trainer flying. She could not tell us how much her hind legs hurt, but her early morning limping, positive rheumatoid factor test, positive mycoplasma tests, and lost weight indicated that something was wrong. It is not just the biggest and heaviest elephants that develop arthritis. Even the youngest elephant in the circus developed arthritis in all four legs, which had been predicted several months earlier by a positive rheumatoid factor blood test.

Degenerative arthritis has been observed in the skeletons of prehistoric woolly mammoths and continues to remain a problem today in many animals, although not readily observed. Elephants remain a mystery and are seriously threatened. We found that many elephants were infected with their own unique species of mycoplasmas. One elephant whose hind legs finally gave out and could no longer stand had to be euthanized. An autopsy revealed extensive destruction of many internal organs in addition to the arthritis. This is not unlike many rheumatoid patients who develop progressive pathology of their internal organs that leads to their death. Learning to live with arthritis may be the only medicine available for some animals. For humans, however, learning all about their disease should help doctors find better medicines and answers for arthritis.

Chapter V
Searching For The Cause To Find The Cure

Not long ago, arthritis and many rheumatoid diseases were thought to be the inevitable results of aging or wear and tear, particularly osteoarthritis, and thus provided little incentive toward searching for causes and cures. Like many other chronic disorders that exhibit a wide variety of symptoms, they seem to present a disease for all seasons and for all people, both young and old, and especially the female, once thought to be the weaker sex.

Those searching for the probable causes, mechanisms, and contributing factors in rheumatoid diseases seem to have been riding a merry-go-round and hoping that the brass ring or magic bullet would fall into their hands. Many investigations have failed to reach out in new and uncharted directions. In spite of many claims, the treatment of rheumatoid diseases has made slow and oftentimes reverse progress with false hopes and promises. Scientists seem to know a lot about the many symptoms and ramifications of the diseases, but the causes remain unknown.

The search for the cause of rheumatoid inflammation requires a determination of the initial onset of the disease even before it reaches the surface and is first diagnosed. We need to know what sequence of factors and conditions preceded the inflammatory symptoms. We can safely rule out aging or wear and tear as the primary cause in rheumatoid arthritis. Even though it is more prevalent in the elderly, children and even infants are also susceptible.

Does physical or mental stress play a role in the initiation of rheumatoid arthritis? If the release of adrenalin or other hormones activate a suppressed or latent inflammatory mechanism, what is the mechanism? Although most people are subjected to stressful situations during their life, they do not always develop rheumatoid arthritis. The Supreme Court has ruled out stress as an occupational hazard. In some people with certain predisposing conditions, the metabolic imbalance from stress can lead to chronic and life-threatening disorders, such as heart disease, stroke, and rheumatoid arthritis.

Finding cortisone from pigs' adrenal glands to act as a potent anti-inflammatory agent for controlling rheumatoid arthritis symptoms, led to the belief or theory that it was caused by a hormonal deficiency. Although some doctors still champion hormonal therapy (discussed in the following chapter), the hormonal and metabolic deficiency theories of cause have apparently lost favor. The range of usefulness of steroids is enormous and even life saving, especially as immunosuppressants, although they are still complicated and dangerous, especially when used excessively.

The potential role of a metabolic cause of rheumatoid diseases, as widely demonstrated in gout, was demonstrated by the establishment of the first Arthritis and Metabolic Institute as part of NIH. Although arthritis now essentially has its own separate institute, the National Institute of Arthritis and Musculoskeletal and Skin Diseases (NIAMSD), the currently accepted belief that the cause is an immunologic disorder of infectious causes would perhaps indicate that it would be more appropriate in the National Institute of Allergy and Infectious Diseases. Because rheumatoid arthritis is also being classified as a collagen vascular and connective tissue disorder that affects the blood vessels, eyes, kidney, heart, lungs, elderly, and infants, all of the institutes at NIH could and perhaps should be searching for the causes and cures of rheumatoid diseases. In fact, the National Institute of Dental Research has paved the way for many advances in arthritis knowledge and treatment.

Pure and basic scientific research has evaluated one factor or one variable at a time, even though humans and experimental animals are comprised of millions if not an infinite number of variables, both internal and external. Recognizing these variables, especially in the complex human host, has placed great weight and emphasis on the predictability of biostatistical analysis. For example, focusing on obesity as a cause of osteoarthritis fails to recognize the loss of or inadequate muscle support. The contribution of muscle fatigue and weakness to arthritis is dependent upon the much acclaimed and publicized exercise requirement of use it or lose it. This in turn is fundamentally dependent upon the vascular blood supply to the muscles, nerves, and other tissues. If anything interferes with the quantity (flow) or quality (composition) of the blood supply, muscle weakness and atrophy will result in joint erosion and pain, together with the damaging effects on other surrounding tissues.

The improper or inadequate supply of essential metabolic nutrients in one's diet or resulting from some gastrointestinal disorder would certainly be a contributing factor to muscle fatigue and weakness and consequently joint damage. The highly vascular joints, much like the brain, eyes, and kidneys, are highly dependent upon the blood supply for adequate oxygen and essential metabolites and thus are also at greater risk for exposure to and deposition of inflammatory toxic and infectious agents.

The probability of researchers identifying any one factor as the contributing cause of rheumatoid arthritis, osteoarthritis, or any of the hundreds of rheumatoid disorders will require a very large computer. Trying to program and analyze the diverse eating habits of Americans would be more difficult than breaking the astronomical genetic code, which at least is relatively constant for humans.

Patients are told that no dieting can cure arthritis while also being told that it is important to eat a healthy, balanced diet. The problem here is determining what constitutes a healthy balanced diet for patients with rheumatoid disorders. Are low-cholesterol and low-salt diets good or bad for arthritics? If a fat-free vegetarian diet reduces heart disease, what does it do for rheumatoid arthritis? What about zinc, copper, or amino acids that have been tested with variable results? What would be the results if they were tested in combination with other elements or substances? One of the most powerful and safest anti-inflammatory agents is the combination of zinc and copper on a protein molecule, a natural product known as superoxide dismutase, an enzyme produced by red blood cells and many vegetables. This is another reason why anemic rheumatoid arthritis patients with low red blood cells have a problem controlling inflammation.

Thus we may ask whether some foods contribute to the cause or possible cure of arthritis. Of course cooking and digesting foods also determine how healthy and beneficial they are and whether they are deficient in some essential element. How do we know that some foods or a vitamin deficiency cannot cause or at least contribute to the severity of arthritis? Several vitamins have recently been promoted to decrease inflammation and thus improve arthritis. Vitamins A (betacarotene), C (ascorbic acid), and E (alphatocopherol), as well as aspirin, are all known to have anti-oxidant activity that can neutralize the excessive cellular oxidation causing the inflammation and pain. When combined with certain metal elements (copper, zinc, and selenium), these vitamins have even greater anti-inflammatory activity. For example, veterinarians have used selenium and vitamin E to control inflammation in arthritic animals and are especially careful to obtain feeds with trace elements. The therapeutic uses of these and other chemicals will be discussed further in following chapters.

Except for gout, there is very little evidence to support a vitamin or dietary deficiency as a cause of arthritis. However, allergies to various foods can enhance or compound the development and expression of rheumatoid and other immunologic disorders, especially those in the delayed-type hypersensitivity arena. Do not be taken in by broad claims that certain foods can cure, heal, or cause arthritis.

Can Arthritis Be Inherited?
The U.S. Public Health Service has reported that a defective gene was found to be the cause of osteoarthritis. Apparently, this is a rare defect not found in all osteoarthritic patients. A genetic or inherited link to arthritis has been heralded on several other occasions only to result in greater anguish by countless millions who fear inheriting the dreaded disease. Unlike the inherited sickle cell anemia, which

carries a destructive genetic expression, patients with chronic and progressive disorders, such as rheumatoid arthritis, diabetes, heart disease, multiple sclerosis, and Alzheimer's, carry an abundance of certain cell surface markers or receptor sites for the causative agents. Fortunately, many other people who carry these same cell surface markers or genotypes have avoided or are protected from the causative agents and contributing factors and thus manage to live free of these so-called genetic or familial disorders. Conversely, the expression of these inheritable disorders in the absence of specific genotypes or cell markers further indicates the primary role of a causative agent and other contributing factors.

If the predominance of female susceptibility to the rheumatoid disorders was determined by the sex-linked genes on the X chromosome that are inherited from the mother, these disorders would occur much more often in males as a recessive sex-linked phenotype, such as color blindness, and hemophilia. Male and female hormones that are genetically controlled can modulate activity of autosomal genes but are not causative.

Back in the 1950s, when the rheumatoid factor, an antibody that developed against the patient's own antibodies, was a suspected cause of rheumatoid arthritis, a doctor transfused the rheumatoid factor positive blood from a patient into a healthy volunteer. Apparently, no symptoms of rheumatoid arthritis developed, and further trials were discontinued. The autoimmune rheumatoid factor is now known to be the result and not the primary cause of rheumatoid arthritis, although it can still contribute to the overall disease mechanism in most (80%) patients.

Investigators, thinking of possible hormonal action and having observed that some female patients appeared to go into remission during pregnancy, transfused the blood from a pregnant patient into a rheumatoid arthritis patient with active arthritis without observing any appreciable benefit. The benefits of hormone therapy are not a replacement, as once thought, but the result of regulating immunologic and other disease mechanisms. Although female estrogen hormone therapy may provide some relief in rheumatoid diseases, its addition does not explain or support the greater incidence in female patients, both young and postmenopausal. Estrogen therapy, acting like an immunosuppressant, could also make females more receptive or reactive to infectious agents. Thus we are still left wondering what causes females, especially of child-bearing age, to have a much greater incidence of rheumatoid diseases than do males.

If rheumatoid arthritis is caused by some infectious agent, what are the risks of blood transfusions from an unsuspected and symptom-free donor? Fortunately, people on medications or with active arthritis would not be accepted donors. That is a good question.

Where Have Investigators Searched For a Cause?

Although many tedious and extensive searches for a bacterial cause in rheumatoid arthritis patients were undertaken in the 1930s, especially when the streptococcal bacteria were found to be associated with rheumatic fever, they were essentially abandoned except for the more obvious cases of acute infectious or septic arthritis. Perhaps the first real clue about the infectious cause of rheumatoid arthritis in humans came in 1939 when the atypical viral-like bacteria called pleuropneumonia-like organisms, now classified as mycoplasmas, were first reportedly isolated from the exudates and tissue of rheumatic patients. Although investigators had shown that mycoplasmas cause arthritis in mice, rats, chickens, goats, and cows, mycoplasmas had been found in the genitourinary tracts of humans (1932-1934), especially females.

A new direction and turning point came in 1949 at the 7th International Congress on Rheumatic Diseases when the possible relationship of mycoplasmas to articular (joint) disease was reported and discussed. Investigators had already observed the effectiveness of the new antibiotic Aureomycin(the first tetracycline) in non-specific urethritis. Other investigators observed the effectiveness of Aureomycin on the mycoplasma induced rat arthritis that was comparable to that obtained by the currently used gold salts. With this knowledge of tetracycline's greater safety and effectiveness than that of gold salts, the direction was clear to test the effect of Aureomycin treatment in patients with a variety of rheumatic diseases.

Reporting on the first successful response to tetracycline in 17 patients, Brown and coworkers concluded in 1949 that only a prolonged clinical trial would determine the therapeutic usefulness

48

and establish the possible relationship of mycoplasmas to articular diseases. Having obtained one of the first NIH research grants (1950), our arthritis research unit reported in 1951 that the rheumatoid disease mechanism was more the result of an immunologic reaction of the antigen (mycoplasma) and its antibody immune complex and not the typical infectious and transmissible disease process.

A few years later (1955), our research unit took this mechanistic approach another step forward when we first reported that mycoplasmas, unlike most infectious agents (bacteria and viruses), could live symbiotically in tissue cell cultures without destroying the tissue cells. Furthermore, this most critical observation, which has been confirmed in many other laboratories, demonstrated the firm and irreversible mycoplasma attachment to tissue cells. This in vitro (test tube) model explained why it would be difficult to isolate mycoplasmas from the patient's tissues and thus demonstrate a cause and effect relationship.

The almost irreversible tissue binding of mycoplasmas has been amply demonstrated in animal models (mice, rats, and pigs). After producing arthritis, the injected mycoplasmas could no longer be isolated from the arthritic animal. This apparently is the same binding mechanism as in humans, especially when the arthritis has become more active. At this later stage, the mycoplasmas not only would be attached to the receptive tissue cells, such as the joint synovium, but also would be complexed and neutralized by their antibodies to form an immune complex, thus producing an inflammatory disease. Mycoplasma infections in both animals and humans are therefore most responsive to tetracycline therapy in the earliest stages, at the onset of symptoms.

Searching the Patients for Clues
In further support of mycoplasmas being a causative agent or antigen, investigators reported at the national Microbiology meeting in 1964 finding a high incidence of mycoplasma antibodies in the blood of rheumatoid arthritis and lupus patients, indicating a previous or current infection. These new observations of mycoplasma infectivity and immunity were further reported in 1965 at the Fifth Interscience Conference on Antimicrobial Agents and

Chemotherapy and the IVth International Congress of Chemotherapy. Of particular importance and perhaps the greatest significance was a finding that females had a much higher incidence (4:1) of mycoplasma antibodies in the hundreds of blood specimens tested from both public and private health clinics. Although still unconfirmed by other investigators, these findings suggest and support a basis for the higher incidence of rheumatoid diseases in females.

Shortly after these reports on mycoplasma infectivity and our pending NIH research grant application on the role of mycoplasmas in rheumatoid diseases, the National Institute of Allergy and Infectious Diseases called a national conference in 1964 to explore the role of infectious agents and immunologic reactions in the genesis of chronic and degenerative diseases. Nothing new or outstanding was proposed, except to agree that evidence of the role of an infectious agent in rheumatoid arthritis was clear. We expressed our view that solving such problems would be more likely if one holds a view of a causative mechanism rather than trying to arrive at a solution categorizing symptoms that are the results and not the cause of the disease.

The view was also expressed that one might have to work with infective agents with human specificity that could not be demonstrated in experimental animals as they may fail to respond immunologically to the human antigen-antibody complex. As already indicated, mycoplasmas are highly species specific, and consequently human strains have not been found in animal models, except for the closely related great apes. It was further suggested that in many of these degenerative diseases, the host conceivably destroys itself by its failure at immunologic self-recognition, the so-called autoimmune disorders. In view of the many unanswered questions, the conferees could not reach a consensus as to the direction and areas of priority research.

Although NIH eventually approved our grant application for half the amount requested, we had already received a research grant from the John A. Hartford Foundation to pursue the role of mycoplasmas in rheumatoid arthritis. Somewhat ironically and most unusual, we had to refuse the NIH award because it would have duplicated support for the same research project. The fact that

50

we received any support was also unusual because a well-known rheumatologist had recently reviewed the possible causes of rheumatoid arthritis and painted a very bleak picture, stating that investigators involved in the study of rheumatic diseases were reluctant to give up their interests and concentrate on what was potentially a dead end.

In addition to the several negative studies cited, further evidence against the role of mycoplasmas in the pathogenesis of rheumatoid arthritis was the lack of any consistent effect of tetracycline therapy on the course of the disease. In spite of these negatives, the 1964 conference review concluded that perhaps the time had arrived for a systematic search for the causative (infectious) agents. This review plus our report may have helped to stimulate the subsequent 1965 NIH conference on infectious agents. Fortunately, we were able to obtain support and pursue our research direction, so that 25 years later (1990) NIH finally initiated a multicenter clinical trial of tetracycline in rheumatoid arthritis patients.

The following year (1966), the National Institute of Arthritis and Metabolic Diseases (now NIAMSD) held a national conference on "The Relationship of Mycoplasmas to Rheumatoid Arthritis and Related Diseases" (PHS publication No. 1523). We were invited to participate along with 40 other experienced investigators in this area. The foreword of the conference proceedings states, "The formerly used synonym of rheumatoid arthritis, 'chronic infectious arthritis,' testifies to the belief long held by clinicians, that an infectious agent may be linked with the etiology of this disease. Although all attempts to prove such a relationship have been unsuccessful to date, there has been a renewal of interest in the question during the last few years. This has followed the development of new microbiologic knowledge and techniques. One such area of particular promise is that of the relationship of the mycoplasma to RA in man and to a naturally occurring arthritic disease in swine resembling RA." It also states, "The increasing interest of investigators in the mycoplasma and the rapid development of mycoplasma-related research findings, and the many pitfalls to be encountered in the work, made it essential that a group of knowledgeable investigators be brought together

51

not only to exchange information but to critically examine the present evidence of a relationship to RA and to stimulate further research. It was equally essential that the deliberations at the conference be made available to the entire research community, since the information has wide applicability."

The proceedings made it clear that at that time human mycoplasma infection had not been definitely linked to rheumatoid arthritis. It also abundantly illustrated the need for more study of the relationship while pointing out the many problems that would have to be solved in relating the disorder to any potential external agent.

The general consensus from the two days of extensive coverage and discussion was that cooperative studies among the various institutions and laboratories were essential to cover such a diverse subject. Many agreed that much more had to be learned about mycoplasmas before they could be related to the very diffuse and even more ill-defined rheumatoid diseases. A question was raised at the conference as to whether apes get any of these diseases or whether anybody had isolated a mycoplasma from them. Someone also stated that if a primate model could be found we would be well ahead of the game. This question was answered by our staff 3 years later, as already discussed. Finding a true animal model of human arthritis, especially when it was successfully tested and treated in several other arthritic gorillas, sparked great interest among researchers and clinicians along with a greater demand for mycoplasma identification and a simplified tetracycline (antibiotic) therapy.

Searching for New Directions in Arthritis
Where has arthritis research been going during the past 25 years (1947-1972), and where should it go over the next 5 years (1972-1977)? To get answers to these questions and set new directions, the Arthritis Foundation convened a blue-ribbon committee of leading researchers in 1972. The committee reported that a breakthrough seemed imminent and the immediate future in arthritis research was promising. The report stated that it was unlikely that we could be able to develop a genuinely effective treatment until the causes were clearly understood. That was 24 years ago.

In addition to increased long-term funding, one of the principal recommendations of the committee was that further study in arthritis research should be directed toward the identification of a possible viral or other infectious agent. Although mycoplasmas, a well-known cause of arthritis in animals, were not even mentioned, the committee did emphasize that the identification of an infectious cause of arthritis would result in one of the biggest payoffs in research. The committee failed to even refer to the mycoplasma arthritis animal models (pigs and gorillas) recently reported by NIH and our laboratory.

The other direction recommended was pinpointing the involvement of the immune system in the chain reaction process of rheumatoid arthritis. The committee stated that major efforts should be directed at clarifying the precise mechanisms for localization of immune complexes (antigen and antibody) in the small blood vessels and kidneys that result in blockage with renal failure and vascular injury. Although it was not mentioned in the committee's report, our laboratory had reported some 20 years earlier on "A Study of the Antigen-Antibody Mechanism in Rheumatic Diseases" (Amer. J. Med. Sci., 221, 1951). Mycoplasma, the infectious antigen, when complexed with its antibody, was the suspected irritant responsible for causing the inflammatory arthritic damage. However, it was not until 1986 that we were able to isolate the immune complex from the rheumatoid arthritis patient's joint fluid and blood and identify the mycoplasma antigen as a component.

The third recommendation was the clarification of the inflammation mechanisms, the first major manifestation of the most serious forms of arthritis. Actually, it is the unseen immune responses that set off the inflammatory responses. The committee noted that particular emphasis should be placed on clarifying the role of enzymes (metabolic digesters) responsible for the destruction of cartilage and other collagenous tissues. This activation and release of digestive enzymes is comparable to the stomach's response to the ingestion of food. Usually the more altered or cooked the food is, the better it is digested by the enzymes. Thus therapy should be directed toward eliminating the infective irritant and also inhibiting the tissue destructive enzymes, such as collagenase. Now 20 years later, NIH has initiated clinically testing the inhibiting effects of tetracycline therapy on the inflammatory enzyme collagenase, which destroys the cartilage, blood vessels, and other tissues in rheumatoid arthritis patients.

The release or activation of the destructive enzyme collagenase, like other digestive enzymes is the result of an irritant, such as an immune complex, that calls into play the body's attempt to destroy the offending irritant. If gone unchecked, the resulting inflammation and destroyed tissues can themselves become an irritant and thus prolong the disease activity. However, the cyclic nature of rheumatoid arthritis, with its peaks and valleys, good days and bad days, certainly suggests the persistence of a latent irritant, such as mycoplasmas, and not a one-shot triggering mechanism, as some investigators have searched for. Unfortunately, the recent NIH clinical trial of the minocycline antibiotic completely failed to look for mycoplasmas or any infectious agent in rheumatoid patients even though frequently recommended.

National Arthritis Act
How many arthritis patients have heard about the National Arthritis Act of 1975? What was it supposed to accomplish and what has it accomplished? With many hundreds of millions of dollars invested in the act, patients are still being told 18 years later that the causes and cures of the rheumatoid diseases are still unknown. Patients are still asking why they have arthritis. With the Arthritis Foundation reporting one million additional arthritis patients each year, it would appear that the very costly Arthritis Plan has been going in the wrong direction searching for the wrong causes and cures. The Arthritis Foundation's 1972 blue-ribbon committee reported that a breakthrough seemed imminent. Extensive lobbying efforts by patients also sparked massive action and support from the federal government, resulting in the passage of the National Arthritis Act of 1975.

It is interesting to note that in 1973 Senator Cranston of California introduced the proposed legislation that would eventually lead to the National Arthritis Act. Companion legislation was introduced by Congressman Paul Rogers of Florida and cosponsored by Congressman Dr. Tim Lee Carter of Kentucky, who later learned about and successfully used Brown's antibiotic approach to arthritis. Congressional hearings further documented the devastating clinical, social, and economic effects of arthritis on patients and the whole country. They also revealed that this major disease had been seriously neglected by federal and other health agencies, which had been anchored in the erroneous beliefs that arthritis was an inevitable disease of old age and wear and tear.

Broadly, the act covered a number of steps to be taken in developing a long-range plan to combat arthritis. The Secretary of HEW appointed an 18-member National Commission on Arthritis and Related Musculoskeletal Diseases to study the arthritis problem in depth and develop an Arthritis Plan with specific recommendations for action (see DHEW publication No. (NIH) 76-1150). The commission's report was submitted to Congress in April 1976 in several volumes. *Volume I. The Arthritis Plan* was entitled "Arthritis: Out of the Maze." The question today is whether we are any further out of the maze or why has the plan failed. In addition to holding 12 public hearings nationwide and surveying existing arthritis activities, the arthritis commission established six workgroups of consultants for community programs, data collection, education, epidemiology, public policy, and research. Although one of our former staff was a member of the commission, our research unit received no additional support or recognition.

Arthritis Plan
The Arthritis Plan reportedly was a blueprint of the broad strategy for a nationwide attack (with international cooperation) against the many arthritis diseases. The commission stated, "The plan is complex, but so is the problem. There are many forms of the disease, possibly each with a different cause . . . . There is today [1976] no known effective method to prevent any of these types. Although means are available to soften the pain and usually control the crippling in some patients, no cures have been found and no effective method of prevention is known." The basic questions remain: What directions were proposed that could lead to the development of cures and preventative methods? Can you find the cure before finding the cause?

Research was only one of several programs recommended in

the Arthritis Plan, and this was further subdivided into clinical and basic research. In pursuing the unknown cause of rheumatoid arthritis, the commission stated that "Programs should be intensified to determine whether an infectious agent, perhaps a bacteria or virus initiates the immunological events". Recommendation 41 was, "High priority should be given to an intensive search for masked, latent or defective viruses and for slow-acting microorganisms that may play a role in rheumatoid arthritis and related diseases." However, the commission further stated, "While an infectious agent has long been thought to initiate rheumatoid arthritis and related diseases, there is yet no convincing evidence to support this hypothesis." My continuing argument to this frequently used barrier to pursuing the possible or probable cause is that if the evidence was sufficiently convincing to the critics, the problem would be solved and there would be no need for further research.

Fortunately, the commission did report that "In view of the existing evidence for immunological phenomena in maintaining inflammation in the joint lining, the antigen or antigens involved in these reactions should be identified, particularly since the chronicity of the disease indicates that the antigens must be present continuously in the synovial environment . . . . There is also sufficient evidence that the antigen-antibody complexes in the joint fluid and joint tissues of patients with SLE and RA play a major role in the initiation (and persistence) of inflammation." The experts again failed to mention mycoplasmas as a potential target. They also did not refer to our report 25 years earlier (1951) on "A Study of the Antigen-Antibody Mechanism in Rheumatic Diseases."

The frequently recommended search for an initiating infectious agent does not explain the chronicity and progressive nature of rheumatoid disorders with ups and downs, good days and bad days. The failure of investigators to consistently isolate any viable infectious agents from rheumatoid arthritis patients not only has discouraged funding of further research but also has applied peer pressure to refute and criticize the validity of those investigators who have obtained positive reports. However, the door could not be shut tight in view of the fact that the experimental arthritis produced in animal models by the injection of mycoplasmas

56

continued long after the mycoplasmas were no longer isolated. Further, mycoplasmas have been detected in tissue cells by chemical means even though they remained nonisolable. The skeptics have kept the door ajar in case new or better techniques would make isolation of the infectious agents possible.

National Arthritis Advisory Board

One of the major recommendations made by the arthritis commission was for the Secretary of HEW to appoint a National Arthritis Advisory Board (NAAB) to provide broad policy guidance and ensure public accountability for actions taken on behalf of the Arthritis Plan. NAAB would replace the commission and appoint working committees and consultants to develop and implement the Arthritis Plan in an advisory capacity to the Secretary of HEW and the Director of NIH. Thus when Congress requested NIH to report on the current research on mycoplasmas and arthritis, NIH requested the NAAB to provide it with a report. NAAB also would make recommendations to the National Arthritis Council of NIH on the research relevance of grant applications seeking support under the act and judged by the peer review groups to be meritorious. Thus the act gave NAAB the control and responsibility of research direction.

The commission also recommended that a separate Arthritis Institute (NIAMSD) should be created at NIH to lead the national effort against arthritis and allied disorders. After extensive lobbying efforts by the Arthritis Foundation and others (not our Institute), Congress approved and funded many millions more to establish a separate Arthritis Institute 10 years later in 1985. Needless to say, the causes and cures of rheumatoid disorders remain unknown. The question still remains, why, especially when Congress has increased the support for arthritis more than 15-fold, from $13 million a year in 1975 to over $200 million in 1992.

Tracking the Infectious Cause of Rheumatoid Diseases

An extensive review of all the studies done to identify an infectious cause of rheumatoid arthritis would fill many library shelves and is beyond the scope of this report. For example, one doctor and her coworkers in Sweden have for more than four decades focused their investigations on the infectious cause of rheumatoid arthritis. More recently, their attention was focused on a streptococcal bacteria (not the strain causing rheumatic fever) that was found in pasteurized milk as the primary cause. Unfortunately, they were unable to show how antibiotics could eradicate both the bacteria and rheumatoid arthritis, and others failed to duplicate their results.

Several investigators have been tracking viruses that are associated with rheumatoid arthritis patients, making them suspected causes. However, like mycoplasmas and bacteria, the viruses or their antibodies can usually be found in both patients and the asymptomatic controls. Some theorize that one virus could alter the genetic DNA of cells, making the cells susceptible to another agent. Such a multiple agent theory is now being investigated in AIDS, where an associated strain of mycoplasmas is suspected of helping the HIV virus to knock out the patient's white cell immunity. This theory is not too far fetched, as most viruses, characterized by killing of tissue cells, can be either helped or hindered by the presence of some mycoplasmas.

As our laboratory first reported, mycoplasmas, unlike most viruses, live on cells but do not kill the tissue cells. Thus mycoplasmas would fit the requirement of a latent or inactive foreign agent. The cause of the immune defect in rheumatoid arthritis patients must be an unusual type of virus—one that does not kill host cells in culture or trigger the production of high levels of antibodies, which typically signals the presence of a virus. The low levels of mycoplasmal antibodies that we have found in rheumatoid arthritis patients have been cited by one expert immunologist as indicating mycoplasma's nonfunctioning role. Unfortunately, some microbiologists still think of mycoplasmas in terms of bacteria or virus properties, which usually results in their trying to fit square pegs in round holes.

A group of investigators in Salt Lake City, searching for the infectious cause of rheumatoid arthritis, tested groups of rheumatoid and nonrheumatoid patients for evidence of present or past infections with mycoplasmas. Using two immunologic test procedures for mycoplasma antibodies, no evidence was found for an association of rheumatoid arthritis patients with the presence of antibodies against any of the four mycoplasma strains tested. As for the prospect of a mycoplasmal cause of human rheumatoid arthritis, the investigators concluded that in view of their negative data the four mycoplasma species tested do not rank as likely etiologic candidates. A group of researchers in Finland reported finding a very high incidence of mycoplasma antibodies in rheumatoid arthritis patients. The two groups of investigators had used different laboratory tests to detect antibodies to the same mycoplasma species, which could account for their markedly different results and conclusions. Using one test, the results from our laboratory were somewhere in the middle. In view of the divergent results and the great impasse on future research direction, we reported that investigators should take another look at mycoplasmas.

Support for the Infectious Cause of Arthritis

In the past, both the NIH and the Arthritis Foundation reported that the search for causes of rheumatoid arthritis had been narrowed to a disorder of the immune mechanisms triggered by an initial infectious process. A form of arthritis resembling rheumatoid arthritis had been produced in pigs with certain mycoplasma organisms. This provided further evidence for the infectious nature of rheumatoid arthritis. The development of arthritis in pigs also provided a long-needed animal model that should greatly aid research. In 1970, our group reported finding and treating an arthritic gorilla naturally infected with mycoplasmas that was a true animal model of human rheumatoid arthritis.

In 1976 NIH stated that a major thrust of its research would continue to revolve around the likelihood that rheumatoid arthritis is the result of an autoimmune reaction triggered by changes brought about by an infectious agent. Investigators were continuing to search for viral agents, but had not yet found any evidence of a viral trigger.

The Arthritis Foundation stated in their booklet *Basic Facts* (1976) that "the precise cause of RA is not yet known, but enough is known now to tell the scientists what kind of cause to look for. There is reason to suspect that a latent virus or similar organism triggers the inflammation of RA. This hypothesis says that a virus-like organism (not the kind of virus people are familiar with) hibernates harmlessly in the body for long period of time until

59

something activates it. Such an organism can be very difficult to detect because it is hidden in the first place, can become active, and do its dirty work, and disappears again . . . . The exciting and hopeful fact is that experts in arthritis research have begun to find tell-tale traces of such organisms in tissues affected by arthritis-type inflammation. These are the beginning of confirmation for the hypothesis. The answer may not be too far off." The foundation stated in its 1977 annual report that "this cause and effect mechanism has been observed often enough to generate fresh efforts to identify the culprit or culprits in RA in particular. This area has become hotter than ever."

If some infectious agent is widely suspected to be the cause of rheumatoid diseases, whether triggering or sustaining, major support by federal, public, and private health agencies to identify the causative mechanism should be the number one priority research item. In fact, both an Arthritis Foundation committee and the HEW commission on arthritis have listed the identification of a possible infectious agent as their first recommendation. The foundation stated in 1972 that "Today's therapy for rheumatoid disease represents the sort of halfway, stopgap measure for palliation of symptoms . . . . It is unlikely that a genuinely effective treatment will be developed either for prevention or cure until the underlying mechanisms are clearly understood."

Five years later, in its 1978 annual report, the foundation concluded that "so far the major risk factor is infection" and then stated that "after many years of research no concrete evidence exists that infection is a risk factor in arthritis." One investigator explained it best: "This has been negative so far but part of the reason may be that we are looking for the wrong bug."

Patients Go to Congress for Help
The role of Congress in determining research direction can be and has been very substantial. As it should be, when the people speak, Congress listens and sometimes acts. As the result of several arthritic constituents reporting to their Congressman Berkley Bedell of Iowa on the successful arthritis treatment they had received, Brown was asked to testify before the House Appropriations Subcommittee about his treatment program and

60

the importance of funds to continue our research. This testimony was published in the *Congressional Record* April 1, 1982 (E1447). As a result of this and other patients' testimony, the House of representatives in September 1982 stated in Report No. 97-894 that "The Committee has been approached by persuasive advocates for the antimycoplasma approach to the treatment of RA. The Committee requests that the NIH make a careful examination of the state of the art of this approach and report to it on the basic research undertaken and presently underway on this method of treatment."

The Senate Appropriations Subcommittee reported on December 8, 1982, in S14144 that "The Committee wishes to be kept apprised of the Institute's (NIH) research into mycoplasma related causes of RA. The committee expects the Institute to examine relevant clinical data and report back within the year its assessment of whatever lines of inquiry may be suggested. Such a review should take into account the possible importance of duration of treatment as a variable in evaluating the mycoplasma perspective."

In response to the Senate's request, NIH asked the National Arthritis Advisory Board (NAAB) to review and make recommendations concerning mycoplasma research. After considering the scientific evidence in both technical reports, the NIH concurred with NAAB's finding and recommendations for future research. Both reports stated that the available scientific evidence was not sufficient to warrant a large-scale, costly clinical trial of antimycoplasma (tetracycline) therapy in rheumatoid arthritis. The NIH report was submitted to the Senate on July 23, 1984, by the Assistant Secretary for Management and Budget in the Department of Health and Human Services (formerly HEW). The NIH report also concluded that the scientific evidence did not support the rationale for using antibiotics in rheumatoid arthritis on a long-term basis.

As for future directions, both the NAAB expert research panel and NIH review recommended two sequential clinical studies, which would be far more costly, in addition to continued mycoplasma-induced arthritis in animal models. The first study was to test for mycoplasmas in joint tissue (synovium) specimens from a large number of rheumatoid arthritis patients and also biopsy tissue samples from another 100 subjects with nonrheumatic chronic arthritis. NIH has reportedly been making plans to initiate this highly unethical and costly project. In the second part of the proposed study, if the biopsy results were positive for mycoplasmas in a sufficiently large number of patients with rheumatoid arthritis, the NAAB expert panel recommended that NIH consider a specific double-blind controlled study of antimycoplasma (tetracycline) therapy in the mycoplasma-positive patients.

The report by the NAAB expert panel stated: "It appears that RA is a disorder involving multiple causative factors. It also seems likely that if mycoplasmas can cause RA it is probable that in only a small percentage of RA petients would mycoplasmas be involved etiologically . . . . Thus a double-blind study only of patients proven to have mycoplasma infection in their joints will be the only way to link antimycoplasma (tetracycline) therapy with efficacy in the complex and heterogenous RA." Actually, the proposed study by NAAB would be an attempt to evaluate a causative role of mycoplasmas in rheumatoid arthritis and certainly not the way to determine the efficacy of tetracycline therapy.

In their report to NIH, the NAAB expert panel also stated that "Because we know that mycoplasmas can cause arthritis in many animals, and because we know that they do cause acute and chronic disease in humans (in lungs and genitourinary tract) we must take seriously the possibility they cause arthritis in humans." What NAAB did not report was that tetracyclines are frequently the antimycoplasma drug used by veterinarians in treating arthritic animals. The NAAB experts should have consulted the Excerpta Medica International Abstracting Service that lists "Mycoplasmic Arthritis" in Section 31, suggesting that mycoplasmas *do* cause arthritis in humans.

Of far greater concern, was why the NAAB expert panel did not consult with the originators and strongest advocates of the antimycoplasma therapy. The panel also did not visit our clinic and ask to review the patients' charts or any other yet unpublished data. As described in the following chapters, both the NIH and the NAAB reports appeared to be negative responses to the paper that we presented in 1981 at the International Rheumatology Congress, which received extensive publicity.

Other Sources of Research Direction

Apparently the NAAB expert panel was not aware of the combined NIH clinical staff conference on "Rheumatoid Arthritis: Evolving Concepts of Pathogenesis & Treatment," which was held on October 13, 1983, and published in the *Annals of Internal Medicine* in 1984.

Besides the high and costly incidence of rheumatoid arthritis another good reason for holding the conference was that "the cause of the disease is still unknown and its treatment is very unsatisfactory." In one report, a rheumatologist listed the possible factors that promote inflammation in rheumatoid joints. The first four causes listed were (1) the deposition of immune complexes, (2) the persistence of mycoplasmas, (3) a chronic viral infection, and (4) the deposition of bacterial cell walls or debris. Rheumatoid arthritis is often referred to as an immune complex disease because of the frequent occurrence of immune complexes (antibody + antigen) in the patient's blood. Thus 2, 3, or 4 could also be part of 1, the immune complex. What is perplexing is that the amount of immune complex circulating in the blood does not always correspond with the disease activity. Consequently, one must recognize that, like in lupus where the immune complex is found attached to the kidney cells, in rheumatoid arthritis the complex must have to attach to the synovial joint tissue cells in order to be a localized and persistent inflammatory irritant. In fact, we must now think in terms of a mycoplasma immune complex capable of attaching to specific cells of most any tissue, including heart, lung, brain, muscles, blood, and pancreas. This is where genetics determines who gets what, when, and where.

In the World Health Organization's 1977 technical report 606 "The Role of Immune complexes in Diseases," rheumatoid arthritis is described as being associated with immune complexes involving immunoglobulin antigens. Although the immune complexes have not been shown unequivocally to cause any of the features of rheumatoid arthritis, they remain the most likely candidates for a number of the disease features. Thus other inflammatory tissue lesions such as rheumatoid pericarditis (heart) and pleuritis (lung) associated with immune complexes have many resemblances to those in the joints (synovitis). Such thinking would lead us in one research direction, and that is to identify the infectious antigen component in the immune complexes. Using new techniques, we examined the immune complexes from rheumatoid patients and reported finding mycoplasma antigens for the first time.

American Rheumatism Association

The American Rheumatism Association (ARA), now the American College of Rheumatology (ACR), is the world's largest professional organization of physicians and scientists dedicated to providing leadership in rheumatology research, education, and patient care. Rheumatologists are doctors who specialize in the care of people with arthritis, diseases of the immune system, and other disorders that cause pain and inflammation in the joints, muscles and bones. Perhaps arthritis patients should ask why the ARA leadership has not found the cause and the cure in the past 40 years.

When Brown's book *The Road Back, Rheumatoid Arthritis —Its Cause and Its Treatment* was published in April 1988 and receiving extensive attention, the ARA issued a fact sheet in an attempt to discredit the book's contents and hence Brown's 50 years of clinical research into the cause and treatment of rheumatoid arthritis. The ARA completely agreed with the earlier NAAB and NIH reports that there was no sound evidence for a relationshp between mycoplasma infection and the development of rheumatoid arthritis. As the leaders of rheumatology research, the ARA should know that mycoplasmas cause arthritis in both animals and humans. Whether the arthritis develops into rheumatoid arthritis or any one of the hundred different forms of rheumatoid diseases still remains our best target. The ARA did state that "It is possible that mycoplasmas could cause RA, but there are no direct confirmations of this hypothesis." The ARA further discounted our reports on antimycoplasma agents (i.e., tetracyclines) being effective in the treatment of rheumatoid arthritis as "not documented by objective criteria and are not sufficient to warrant a broad-scale study of these drugs in RA (1988)."

Apparently sufficient objective criteria were located by the ARA, as one year later NIH launched a costly, multicenter, long-term clinical trial of tetracycline's (minocycline) effectiveness in rheumatoid arthritis. In 1987, having recently found for the first time mycoplasmal antigens in the immune complexes from rheumatoid arthritis patients, we submitted an abstract of these new key findings to the ARA for presentation at its national meeting. (These results were later published in 1989 in The Annals of Allergy.) Since most current research was now pointing in the direction of immune complexes, it seemed unusual that the ARA did not accept our report and admit this most significant new evidence of mycoplasma's role in rheumatoid arthritis.

Workshop on the Infectious Cause of Early Arthritis

A Workshop on the Infectious Cause of Early Arthritis was called by the director of the Arthritis Institute at NIH in November 1985, which was partially responsive to the reports requested by Congress. A score of investigators interested in the possible viral, bacterial, and mycoplasmal cause of arthritis presented their ideas on how, where, and when to search for infectious agents. Many ideas and suggestions, including our own, were presented. Unfortunately, there was no unified consensus on who would do what, especially when the pending funding was nebulous. Of course the big question was how early is early and the need to exclude the juveniles that might harbor a latent agent. As the animal models had frequently demonstrated, the recovery or isolation of mycoplasmas could be made only in the earliest signs of arthritis, which may take a different onset and course in humans. This failure to isolate viable microorganisms from the inflamed tissues has convinced some investigators that the agent is persisting as a neutralized complex and/or tightly bound to tissue cells.

We know that mycoplasmas have a high affinity to the cells in tissue cultures, frequently causing researchers to believe they are absent when they resist isolation. Recently, ultrasensitive and costly techniques have been developed that now make it possible to detect trace amounts of mycoplasmas and other agents in diseased tissues. As previously noted, even finding a microbial agent in the diseased tissue does not alone prove that it is the cause as it could also be an innocent bystander or even a cofactor.

Perhaps another more direct way of pinning down the causal agent, short of infecting human volunteers or the great apes, would be to find an effective therapeutic drug that cures or reduces disease activity and compare the activity with the loss of the agent from the patient's tissues. If the safer tetracycline therapy controls rheumatoid arthritis and provides a road back to good health, its widespread usefulness and efficacy should not continue to be withheld while researchers spend many more years looking for the infectious cause.

Even though the NAAB recommended that we must take seriously the possibility that mycoplasmas cause rheumatoid arthritis in humans, there has been no serious or concerted effort by NIH or other investigators to pursue this direction until recently. This neglect was further indicated by the absence of any related report at the 1992 biannual meeting of the International Organization of Mycoplasmologists. The interest in mycoplasmas as human pathogens increased recently after investigators discovered a new mycoplasma strain in AIDS patients. The question now remains whether mycoplasmas are a cofactor with the HIV virus in the cause of AIDS, while their role in human rheumatoid arthritis remains unsolved on the so-called drawing board.

International League Against Rheumatism
At the 1989 International Congress of Rheumatology in Brazil, the continuing search for the cause of rheumatoid arthritis was reported as one of several related autoimmune diseases. The search for a cause of rheumatoid arthritis still centers today, as it did at the 1985 ILAR meeting, on microbial agents that can stimulate immune responses in specific (not normal) individuals.

One theory still persists that an immune reaction to bacterial cell wall components initiates arthritis in susceptible animals. However, neither the bacteria nor the cell wall components (peptidoglycans) have been found in the synovial tissues of rheumatoid arthritis patients as they have in animal models. If bacteria cell walls were the cause of rheumatoid arthritis, then penicillin therapy, which inhibits cell wall synthesis, should stop and even prevent rheumatoid arthritis but does not.

Another theory demonstrated in an animal model is that the injection of complete Freund's adjuvant (a suspension of bacterial Tb components in mineral oil) can cause the development of

66

arthritis in susceptible strains of rats. The only question here is what infectious agent naturally acts like an adjuvant in humans, certainly not Tb in oil.

Another possible infectious cause of rheumatoid arthritis still considered by some is the Epstein-Barr virus (EBV), which like mycoplasmas is present in most adults. Also like mycoplasmas, tissue mimicries have been identified in EBV. Therefore, if it is the cause of rheumatoid arthritis, it will be through autoimmunity reaction with specific host tissues. The question here is what effect the arthritis drugs—gold salts, plaquenil, tetracycline, and especially the immunosuppressants—have on EBV in the rheumatoid patients. Even the common bacteria *Proteus mirabilis* was suggested as a possible cause of rheumatoid arthritis. It has been further theorized that a peptide molecule (a small protein) from any of the above organisms would cross-react with the host tissues to induce rheumatoid arthritis.

These theoretical causes of rheumatoid arthritis presented at the 1989 rheumatology Congress are markedly different mechanisms than the one Clark presented at the same Congress. He presented data that showed a new mechanism of mycoplasma's role in rheumatoid and other immunologic disorders. Mycoplasmas could act as a viable antigen carrier (adjuvant), as an immune complex (mycoplasma and antibody), and also as a self-antigen (mycoplasma and tissue antigen) binding and altering specific proteins from patients' tissues.

Examples of mycoplasma's pathoimmunologic mechanism were previously observed by other investigators when mycoplasmas were observed to selectively remove protein antigens from the infected red blood cell membranes. These auto antigens from the red blood cells were found to be associated with the positive serologic cold agglutinin test frequently observed in patients infected with *Mycoplasma pneumoniae* and may also be associated with anemia in other disorders. Another highly relevant example of mycoplasma's specific autoantigen production, at least in vitro, was also finding that mycoplasmas could selectively remove and bind specific protein antigens from the white blood cell membranes. The mycoplasma production of such a white cell autoantigen and the resulting antibody reaction to one's own white cells could be the basic mechanism of several other immunologic disorders.

Although NIH, the NAAB expert panel, and the American Rheumatism Association had all agreed in previous reports that the mycoplasma's role in rheumatoid arthritis should be taken seriously, it was not demonstrated at the 1989 rheumatology Congress. Their total lack of concern was shown by Clark's report being the only one on mycoplasmas in over a thousand presented at the rheumatology Congress. His paper entitled "Mycoplasma Bound IgG Expresses Autoantigenic Antiidiotypic Antibodies" reported in part that many chronic degenerative diseases such as rheumatoid arthritis were suspected of resulting from autoimmune mechanisms of unknown infectious etiology. Although associated with autoantibodies and antigenic mimicry, mycoplasmas had never been shown until then to express autoimmunogens. In addition to the infectious and immune complex reactivity, these results demonstrated a potential role and pathogenic mechanism of mycoplasmas causing conformational changes of bound IgG (immune globulin) that could also apply to other tissue proteins. By producing altered self antigens, mycoplasmas could initiate a variety of human autoimmune disorders (in Am. J. Primatology 24:1991, pp 235-243). This investigation, conducted with rabbits, was able to demonstrate a mechanism whereby mycoplasmas could initiate the production of a rheumatoid factor as an anti-antibody or autoantibody to the host's own IgG immune globulin.

Future Directions to the Cause
The search for the microbial cause of rheumatoid diseases should be directed toward the immune complexes producing inflammatory diseases. Many of the chronic immunologic diseases, such as rheumatoid arthritis, that are attributed to immune complexes are also suspected to be of microbial origin. This suggests that the causative inflammatory agent must exist in the form of a viable but neutralized complex in order to produce a persistent chronic disease. Therefore, neither the separate viable microbial agent nor its free antibodies would be readily associated with disease activity unless attached to the host's tissue cells.

The association of the so-called autoimmune reactivity with the rheumatoid disorders points toward an agent or agents that are also instrumental in eliciting an autoimmune response. Whether the autoantibodies that are directed toward specific host cell components are a primary or secondary cause of the rheumatoid diseases remains to be demonstrated. The fact that mycoplasmas have frequently been associated with autoimmune activity and are known to elicit autoimmune reactivity in animal models should definitely make mycoplasmas the first direction of future investigations, as so often proposed.

To find the answers, the corporations and others making profits from arthritis patients should provide significant support for research directed toward the infectious cause of rheumatoid diseases.

Chapter VI
Searching For A Cure

A rthritis has been known to exist since prehistoric times and for more than 2,000 years been recognized as a clinical entity, following the original clear description of the disease by Hippocrates. Over 5,000 remedies have been devised, and despite the magnitude of the therapeutic efforts and basic research, rheumatoid arthritis still remains the most progressive and destructive disease of unknown cause and cure.

Arthritis is older than civilization and still persists today probably because it is not recognized as a killer disease, even though its many victims die prematurely. Although there may be many reasons for the animal survival instinct in humans, the advent of civilization started when humans not only protected but tried to help each other. It was no longer a survival of the fittest but an increasing concern and recognition for the less fit, as the value of life and living gradually became accepted. Tribal doctors, witch doctors, medicine men, spiritualists, and eventually doctors taking the Hippocratic oath have tried various means to control and stop or eradicate the consumptions of unknown causes. Fortunately, some societies became more concerned and active in saving the lives of the affflicted, especially when Christianity and other religious beliefs began to set higher values on life. Now, looking around at the world's "civilized" nations, one can only wonder and question how high their values of life are. The United States spends considerably more on a standard of living than more populated countries and with substantially increased expenditures every year. The real problem is that our values on life seem to keep going down with the value of the dollar.

Our priorities to save and protect lives at any cost have reached a critical problem that threatens the very lives that are to be protected. Who is in charge? Who is the medicine man today? The Surgeon general, NIH, USPHS, AMA, or ARA? Who is responsible for finding the causes and cures of the many prevalent diseases that continue to kill and cripple? Or who is responsible for failing?

Why, when, and how did today's therapies develop? They were first developed probably based on the mothering instincts of most animals to nurture and protect their offspring and the subsequent family and tribal efforts to survive. We might even suggest that the medicine man or witch doctor provided the first national health care programs in their communities. Perhaps some care was for the preservation of the tribe, some to please the gods, and some for humanitarian reasons. What was important were the various methods of care passed down through the generations over hundreds and thousands of years, which some may consider were the origin and basis of today's medical education system. Even more important were the tribal doctors who for one reason or another made an extra effort to look for stronger medicines. Not many doctors make that extra effort today, although most have taken the Hippocratic oath to save lives. The so-called magic bullets came much later. However, even today, with our very costly high-tech equipment and diagnostic skills, we are still at a loss to explain much of their magic. While some potions may still be brushed off as so much quackery, other scientists are still searching the world's far corners for better magic.

Magic or Miracles

What have we learned from or how do we explain some of the successful therapies from yesterday or today? Were they real or imaginary or a little of both? Through the centuries, the power of religious beliefs and the forceful conviction of the spiritualists seemed to have provided as much relief as the medicine man or medical practitioners. If the patient got better, one could claim that it was a miracle or their magic, while the others attributed it to their medicine. In any case, the experts today still claim that there is no known cure. Then why did those few miracle cases get better while others did not? Was it because some patients were different or because there were different causes untouched by the medicine?

The power of mind over matter can be, has been, and will continue to be one of our more powerful therapeutic weapons. Today's scientists are rediscovering some of the many ways that the brain controls or regulates biological functions. For example, some of our strongest emotions, love, hate, fear, and stress, processed through our brain, evoke hormonal and other biological responses that could improve or worsen disease mechanisms. The power of prayer or of positive thinking could have a substantial impact on the results of therapy. How strongly you hope and pray that the medicine will make you better apparently becomes an unmeasurable aspect of therapeutic effectiveness.

Several years ago, noted writer Norman Cousins described his personal experience in overcoming a life-threatening connective tissue disorder using the powers of the mind in his article *Anatomy of an Illness*. His recovery was attributed to the healing powers of laughter and megadoses of vitamin C. He later went on to test the physiologic basis of the ancient theory that laughter is a good medicine and that the key to coping with a disease is the patients' positive attitudes and control of their emotions. If stress and depression weaken the immune defenses, then the opposites should improve the immune system. There now seems to be a scientific basis for believing that hope, faith, love, and the will to live have a bearing on the outcome of an illness. The teaspoon of sugar that helps the medicine go down still applies. Why does or how does the patient's willful determination to live, to beat the odds, make a difference? In an effort to research the interactions between the brain and the body, medicine has established a new branch of psychoneuroimmunology.

The suffering rheumatoid arthritis patients have two strikes against them as they limp into the doctor's office having lost all hope for a cure and worrying that the next more toxic medication will be the third and final strike. On the other hand, a patient who has been given hope may benefit, if only for a short period, from a nonmedicinal sugar pill known as the placebo effect. Thus a controlled therapeutic trial using a placebo should be evaluated over a sufficiently long period of several months in order to separate and evaluate both the beneficial and toxic side effects. In fact, the Arthritis Foundation and American Rheumatism Association have often critized Brown's tetracycline therapy, attributing his success to a placebo effect of his skilled, confident, and compassionate delivery of health care. They have not explained his successful long-term treatment of both humans and gorillas. Unfortunately, most rheumatologists, having lost the confidence in the magic of available therapies, often wish that they could sneak out their back door when they see a rheumatoid patient enter the office, except for the fact that these patients support their clinics. No disease is more depressing and demoralizing than rheumatoid arthritis, and unless doctors give patients hope and inspiration, their medication will fall short of its goal.

We Have Come a Long Way
Wittingly or unwittingly, physicians have been using antibacterials since history began. Ancient Egyptian physicians recognized the antibacterial properties of certain fermentation products, including beer. They often prescribed the lees that collected in the bottom of ceramic brewing vats as an important emollient in treating infections (circa 2560 B.C.) A plaque from an Egyptian pillar of the eighth dynasty (circa 2160 B.C.) shows a physician dispensing medications masked in beer to the high priest Indy. The medication may or may not have been effective but the beer or its sediment would contain fermentation products that have antibiotic action.

It is now recognized that some of the antibiotic properties could have come from the moldy grain used to make beer. Recently, a research group in Amherst studying osteoporosis in the skeletal remains of villagers living in Sudan dating to 550 A.D. found traces of tetracycline in their bones. The researchers theorized that the most probable source of the tetracycline was the mold-like bacteria called streptomycetes, common in the desert soil of Sudan. It most likely came from the wheat, barley, and millet stored in mud bins. Scientists have long been puzzled by the good health of these

74

We Have Come a Long Way

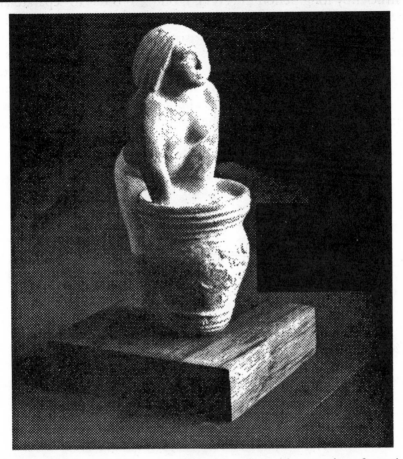

Ancient Egyptian physicians recognized the antibacterial properties of certain fermentation products—beer among them. They often prescribed "yeast of sweet beer" (the lees that collected in the bottom of ceramic brewing vats) as an important emollient in treating boils and infected wounds. The statuette shown here (from the 5th Dynasty, 2560-2420 BC) depicts a woman straining beer mash, made from partially baked, fermented bread dough, into such a vat through a wicker sieve. Original of this tomb figure, in limestone, is in the National Museum, Cairo. Permission to publish the photograph of the servant brewing by Dr. Mohamed Saleh, Director, The Egyptian Museum. Cairo, Egypt.

Antibacterial Therapy - a fact of medicine from time immemorial

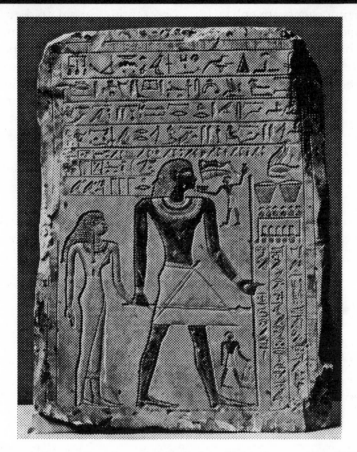

Plaque made from an Egyptian stele (pillar) of the Eighth Dynasty (circa 2160 BC) shows a physician in the act of dispensing medication masked in beer to his patient, the high priest Indy. Behind Indy is his wife, the priestess of goddess Hat-Hor-Mut-Manty. The medication may or may not have been effective, but the beer (or its sediment) would contain fermentation products which have antibiotic (antibacterial) action. Original in New York's Metropolitan Museum. Permission to use the above photograph given by The Metropolitan Museum of Art, Rogers Fund, 1925. (25.2.3) VI-XII Dynasty, (2475-2000 B.C.) Stela of the Count Indy. Painted limestone.

isolated groups who lacked access to modern medicine.

The widespread prescribing of tetracycline in the 1950s led to the discovery of its strong chelating properties with the binding and staining in calcifying tissues and thus found in bones. This most unusual discovery raises questions as to what other naturally occurring agents are enhancing or preventing rheumatoid or other chronic diseases. Will some scientists a hundred years from now find that the high pollen or mold counts in the air we breathe contribute to some form of cancer or even the chronic fatigue syndrome? Perhaps the inhalation of viruses bound to air pollutants, such as cigarette smoke, may be contributing to lung cancer in nonsmokers. In our little known and highly variable environment, we may even find that the ingestion of the popularized so-called natural foods may actually contain unknown environmental ingredients more harmful than the synthetics. The back to nature move may not be available for all people, who now realize that we can not go back to the jungle when our cities become polluted. We have come a long way to achieve greater longevity, but at what expense. What have we accomplished in terms of input versus output? Is modern medicine really worth the cost, and what are the limits?

Spas, Health clubs and Exercise

Some of the earliest forms of physical therapy (exercise) and hydrotherapy are still found in the warm mineral baths and spas throughout southern Europe. These were later developed and promoted in the United States, providing arthritic and polio patients some precious pain-free moments. With the easing of pain and stiffness, patients were now able to move and stretch muscles that were fast becoming wasted and unusable. Even with the introduction of aspirin and other painkillers, physical therapy developed new and more effective forms of active and passive exercises that provided longer periods of comfort and function but rarely a remission. Exercises, together with warm towels and paraffin baths, became key ingredients, especially to maintain muscle strength and a full range of motion. Although some arthritics are able to attend health clubs or massage parlors, nonarthritics seemed to have gotten the message that stronger muscles will protect the joints from wear and tear and thus minimize their chance of developing arthritis. Similarly, developing stronger heart muscles not only protects against heart disease but provides a stronger pump for the all-important blood circulation to maintain healthy joints, nerves, and skin, as well as muscles. The old slogan "use it or lose it" is especially important for the crippled and feeble patients who depend on the passive exercises of their therapist or family to massage and thus stimulate the blood circulation.

Most rheumatic diseases are the result of vascular disorders that limit the blood supply of essential oxygen and nutrients to the joints and other tissues or limit the return and removal of waste products. Maintaining a strong and healthy cardiovascular system is a key ingredient to disease-free good health. Even with an adequate amount of muscle exercise from swimming, walking, aerobics, and other activities, the lungs must still provide sufficient oxygen, the gastrointestinal (GI) tract must provide essential nutrients, and the liver and kidneys must eliminate the toxic waste products in the blood. Early morning stiffness, one of the yardsticks used to measure rheumatoid arthritis is the result of many reactions. When the sleeping or resting muscles slow down metabolic activity, the body temperature drops with lower blood pressure and decreased circulation. With the lowering of body temperature, especially in the hands and feet, the joint fluid becomes more viscous and stiff, like gelatin, until increased activity or a hot shower raises the body's temperature. The early morning stiffness and chronic fatigue could be the result of poor circulation with inadequate oxygen due to anemia, malnutrition, metabolic deficiencies, and limitation of the high-energy molecules consumed by the nonmuscular organs and tissues. The remarkable body functions prioritize energy to the more vital organs. Of course the GI problems associated with rheumatoid arthritis could greatly limit the supply of nutrient energy. This over or under energy production would partially explain the extended periods of fatigue and why some patients are more comfortable where it is warm while others prefer the cooler climate.

Much of the inflammatory activity in rheumatoid arthritis, with heat, swelling, and redness, is largely the result of excessive oxidation in the joints by the white blood cells trying to destroy the irritant. This overactivity would utilize and deprive the body of its energy sources, leading to weakness and atrophy. After many years of joint research, the role of excessive oxidation in causing inflammation and its control has narrowed the search to antioxidant therapy that reduces inflammation and the resulting pain and destruction. Rather than focusing on the cause of the fire or inflammation, most clinicians look for better ways to extinguish the blaze. Unfortunately, the approved extinguishers have failed to control the persistent spark and the progressive destruction.

In the 1930s, doctors were promoting sulfur-containing foods, which were considered reducing agents or antioxidants and seemingly limited the amount of inflammation. When it was learned that a natural fatty acid (arachidonic) was oxidized to form gonadotropin, a pain-causing hormone, attention was shifted to drugs that inhibit the oxidizing enzyme. Thus many of the currently used anti-inflammatory drugs, or so-called NSAIDS, have pain-reducing properties by shutting down the release of enzymes with oxidizing and destructive activity. As many patients have experienced, most medications, like exercises, have individual tolerable or antagonistic levels that must be tailored for maximum benefits. To maintain its biologic chemistry and functions, the human body requires combustible nutrients as well as oxygen. If this oxygen supply to the brain is limited via the blood supply, even for a short time, the brain stops functioning and the whole body stops. On the other hand, inhibition of all the oxidizing enzymes could also shut down the body. The therapeutic objective is to use drugs at minimum or intermittent tolerable doses that partially inhibit the excessive oxidation or fire but still leave the pilot flame burning. A good example is the intermittent or every other day doses of tetracycline that can permanently inhibit the oxidative respiratory enzymes unless the tissues are given a day or two to catch their breath. Therapy directed toward the control and reduction of inflammation is most essential as it could provide a less hostile and optimum environment for other therapies, such as antibiotics, directed toward the causative agent.

Diet as a Cure or a Cause
The Food and Drug Administration (FDA) and the U.S. Public Health Service (USPHS) have now dropped the minimum daily requirement (MDR) of vitamins as apparently there is no concern

for vitamin deficiencies in our nation's dietary habits. Hopefully they are not telling all senior citizens to stop taking their multivitamin pill. Like ultraviolet (UV) rays, vitamins and trace minerals can be over or under utilized. Because vitamins and minerals are readily excreted and not stored, a constant minimal availability is essential for special occasions.

For example, the fat-soluble vitamin D precursor, ergosterol, found in most daily diets (eggs, yeast, milk, and fish oils) requires ultraviolet exposure (irradiation) to be converted to its active form calciferol (D2). Babies who are protected from the sun's UV rays usually receive their vitamin D2 from irradiated formula. However, senior citizens on low-fat and low-cholesterol diets and not able to get sufficient sunshine may become good candidates for osteoporosis with the reduction in calcium utilization and metabolism. In addition to their aching joints, perhaps the attraction to sunshine is the reason why so many northerners retire in the sunshine states. Like everything else, excessive sunshine or vitamins can cause as much damage as benefit. The sun, which provides life and energy to all creatures, does not guarantee freedom from disease and pain, even though its warmth is soothing.

Perhaps the best rule to follow is one of moderation and variety. As yet, there is no perfect food that meets all nutritional requirements and no perfect diet for all. As any good farmer knows, a well-nourished plant or animal is more resistant to diseases but provides no guarantee. Some people believe that special diets or exotic foods benefit arthritis, while others believe that some foods can cause arthritis, especially if they are allergic to them. As the Arthritis Foundation reported in their *Basic Facts* booklet (1976), "If there was a relationship (cause & effect) between diet and arthritis it would have been discovered long ago . . . . The simple fact is: there is no scientific evidence that any food or vitamin deficiency has anything to do with causing arthritis and no evidence that any food or vitamin is effective in treating or 'curing' it, and the truth is vitamins do not help arthritis." Some doctors now take the extreme opposite view, claiming that the proper diet and healthy living can prevent and eliminate arthritis and many other symptoms.

If these are the facts, then why are the vitamins A, C, and E, with antioxidation properties, now being recommended as potential anti-inflammatory therapeutic agents? Like aspirin, they may help to reduce inflammation but certainly are not a cure for the inflammatory rheumatoid diseases. The veterinarians who for years have been treating their arthritic animals with vitamin E and selenium must believe that these dietary components have some medicinal benefits. In zoos and circuses, the caretakers make sure that the hay is not deficient in selenium.

Antioxidants and Anti-inflammatory Therapy

Although it was little known or recognized 40 years ago, one of the major causes of tissue inflammation is now well known and investigated. The culprit known as superoxide is the most active and hottest oxygen molecule prior to its neutralization and combination with hydrogen, resulting in hydrogen peroxide (H_2O_2) and water (H_2O) formation. The amount of potential destructive energy in this radioactive superoxide is comparable to the amount of electrical energy required to split the H_2O molecule. It is a far stronger oxidant than hydrogen peroxide, which can dissolve tissues and microorganisms.

What has superoxide to do with inflammatory arthritis? Although the human body has many biochemical reactions that metabolize and detoxify chemical irritants that are ingested or contacted, it also has many other chemical processes to destroy and remove the infectious and noninfectious agents. A fever and an elevated white blood cell count are some of the early symptoms indicating that an infectious disease is in progress. Usually the more virulent and active the infectious agent (bacteria, virus, mycoplasma), the higher the white blood cell count and the fever. Having detected the foreign intruder, the body starts producing more white blood cells (killer cells) designed to attack and destroy the foreign agent. In order to do this, the white blood cells are equipped with various digestive (proteolytic) and oxidative enzymes. When the irritant is trapped in the joint, an excessive number of white blood cells infiltrate the tissue and rapidly destroy the foreign substances. The excessive localized oxidation by the white blood cells may help to destroy the germs, but the excessive heat and release of destructive proteolytic enzymes, such as collagenase, become over destructive and painful to the surrounding joint tissues. Similar phenomena

81

occur when a boil or an abscess results from a localized infection. With a limited blood supply, the white blood cells and debris accumulate in the confined area, leaving a boil full of sterile pus.

Under normal conditions, with an adequate supply of blood, the red blood cells also carry out their multiple life-sustaining functions. The hemoglobin in red blood cells controls respiration by its adsorption and distribution of oxygen and other gases to and from the tissues. The red blood cells also produce one of the most potent antioxidants in the form of a protein enzyme containing copper and zinc called superoxide dismutase (SOD). As its name suggests, SOD is very active in neutralizing the most irritating superoxide. Thus when white blood cells concentrate in the joints without sufficient fire-extinguishing red blood cells, inflammation results. The SOD enzyme is also found in green vegetables, and some investigators have tested the concentrated enzyme in several inflammatory diseases, including rheumatoid arthritis. Unfortunately, enzymes being proteins are readily inactivated and destroyed in the GI tract, making their oral therapy very limited. Other forms and routes of administration have been tried with variable success. Because of SOD's relative abundance in natural products, with far greater activity than nonsteroidal anti-inflammatory drugs (NSAIDS), its potential application has never generated sufficient clinical research support. One such potential application of SOD, as demonstrated in experimental animals, was minimizing the damage from excessive x-ray therapy and ionizing radiation that also results from superoxide. Several other potential SOD applications to minimize excessive oxidation and radiation are being investigated.

Aspirin, Still the Number One Anti-inflammatory Therapy
Undoubtedly the most widely used anti-inflammatory and anti-arthritic drug used and still the medication of first choice is aspirin or acetylsalicylic acid. It has been estimated that Americans consume 16,000 tons of aspirin tablets per year, which would represent close to 60 billion pills of arthritis or other strengths. While some arthritics may consume over 1,000 pills a year, there are still many who have avoided the number one pill. Even though aspirin comes in many different forms and is recommended or taken for many ailments and afflictions, it still possesses some deleterious as

well as beneficial effects. Aspirin's multiple actions in various disorders and symptoms, although not considered curative, are still not fully recognized or understood, especially their preventative mechanisms.

The nonsteroidal anti-inflammatory drugs (NSAID) stop pain by inhibiting the oxidative enzyme (prostaglandin H synthase) that converts the common arachidonic fatty acid to the pain-causing prostaglandin hormone. In addition, aspirin has strong chelating or binding properties and can bind copper, zinc, iron, calcium, and many other divalent metal ions. It can also inhibit the metal-containing enzymes and thus alter many cellular functions. As a copper complex, copper-aspirinate can also act catalytically as an antioxidant or anti-inflammatory agent by neutralizing the inflammatory superoxide $(O^-)_2$ (see "Inflammatory Diseases and Copper", Ed. J.R.J. Sorenson, Humana Press, 1982). Unfortunately, limited research support and bad press have curtailed further investigation and clinical trials of these and other metallic compounds, such as selenium, that could result in rheumatoid arthritis patients going off the gold standard. Copper chelates, such as copper-aspirinate, copper-tetracyclinate or even copper-penicillamine, can act like the anti-inflammatory SOD enzyme. As a result, they can also inhibit the primary inflammation reactions that activate the destructive and pain-causing enzymes.

Another critical metalloenzyme, collagenase, which causes the destruction of collagen protein in the joint's connective tissues, is inhibited by tetracycline and other metal-binding, chelating agents. Further research on aspirin, tetracycline, ascorbic acid, and other chelating compounds could greatly expand our knowledge of their diverse, multiple actions. Some doctors have even promoted using a mixture of chelating agents, including vitamin C, for rheumatoid arthritis therapy. Many investigators have championed the cause of vitamin C without understanding its multiple actions.

Penicillamine, one of the so-called disease modifying drugs approved and highly promoted for rheumatoid arthritis therapy and the byproduct of the penicillin antibiotic, is also a copper chelating agent. In fact, one of its approved applications is in Whipple's disease, which is characterized by an excessively high copper blood level. Originally approved as a substitute for gold therapy, pencillamine has more recently been implicated in the initiation or on-set of lupus (SLE). Of particular interest was finding that when complexed with copper, penicillamine also becomes an antimycoplasma agent, which may partially explain some of its thera-peutic effectiveness.

What many investigators seem to have overlooked in their controlled clinical trials of a drug's effectiveness, or toxicity, is that there is no such thing as a single reactive element, or chemical, once it enters the body's complex biological system. The failure to show any significant dietary benefits from zinc, copper, or an amino acid in rheumatoid arthritis patients is because they do not func-tion separately; neither do chelating agents. Furthermore, the ex-cessive concentration of any one of the metabolic components (copper, zinc, vitamins A or C, etc.) could inhibit rather than en-hance a delicately balanced equilibrium reaction. To complicate the reactions further, each patient may respond differently. Even caged rats that are litter mates and the same sex may not respond identically to the same diet. The arthritis-strength aspirins that are buffered with calcium or zinc or enteric coated may have different rates of absorption into the blood and tissues, which do not assure maximum benefits. As long as it reduces inflammation, pain, and swelling and does not irritate your stomach, the rapidity of the re-action is less important.

The acid and alkali, the negative and positive charges, must be balanced for each individual system in order to achieve their optimum or so-called normal healthy condition. Finding the right combination of drugs, as is now currently being investigated, in the right or optimum proportions and at the right time is frequently the problem. Although both gold and copper therapy have been used in rheumatoid arthritis patients, the less reactive gold salts had lower toxicity than the highly reactive copper salts. Even though copper is a natural and essential biological component, it failed in favor of the unnatural and less active gold. Like gold, aspirin is extremely insoluble and usually requires a carrier to help it reach its target. The ionic copper salt and other metals differ in their elec-tron scavenging or antioxidant/anti-inflammatory activity, with cop-per one of the most active and gold one of the least.

Proven and Unproven Treatments

When the NSAIDS fail, there are several other usually more toxic drugs available that may provide additional relief for some patients. These drugs, called disease-modifying antirheumatic drugs (DMARS,) can help some patients whose arthritis persists and remains active with swollen and inflamed joints. These DMAR drugs, which do not cure rheumatoid arthritis and can have many adverse side effects, include gold salts, D-penicillamine, antimalarials, and the more recent methotrexate, a former cancer drug that also has immunosuppressive activity. Usually the more potent immunosuppressing drugs, like cortisone, are used in the more severe and active rheumatoid arthritis patients who have not been controlled by the DMAR drugs. Their toxicity and adverse side effects greatly curtail their usefulness and short-lived benefits, which fall far short of the infectious cause. In fact, the so-called disease-modifying drugs are now reported to not modify the course of rheumatoid arthritis.

The treatment or management of rheumatoid arthritis is of necessity somewhat programmatic and must be adapted to each patient's changing needs with the realization that there is no magic bullet. Most arthritis therapies are empirical and symptomatic, directed toward the suppression and control of inflammation and pain. Other physical efforts are used to maintain function along with the prevention and repair of deformities, such as splinting and surgery. As one noted rheumatologist remarked in 1979, "Although an infectious etiology for rheumatoid arthritis remains attractive, therapy currently accepted as appropriate is not based on an infectious cause." In an article on quackery, the chairman of the Arthritis Foundation's Unproven Remedies Committee reportedly gave a patient a realistic view of accepted treatments by explaining that "their goal is not the eradication of the disease, but maintenance of function. The patient should be encouraged to focus on living a normal life with a tolerable level of pain and discouraged from looking for a cure." With this attitude, many doctors have become discouraged in their search for a cure or a cause. If the Arthritis Foundation's goal is not the eradication of rheumatoid arthritis, whose goal is it?

Although it is not well known or publicized, the currently accepted treatment of rheumatoid arthritis with gold was originally

85

applied in the preantibiotic 1920s and based on the unproven theory when Tb was thought to be the cause. Of course today, patients with Tb or bacterial arthritis are successfully treated with broad spectrum antibiotics and thus far are much better off than the rheumatoid arthritis patients who are still treated with gold. Now 70 years later, rheumatologists are finding that gold therapy does not stop or modify the course of rheumatoid arthritis and becomes an intolerable poison in most patients within 5 years.

When mycoplasmas were found to cause arthritis in mice and rats in the 1930s, it was fortuitous to test and demonstrate the preantibiotic effects of gold on mycoplasma inhibition and hence on the control of arthritis. Although it benefited arthritic mice and rats, veterinarians could not safely use gold on the larger animals (cows, sheep, goats, pigs, etc.) with mycoplasma arthritis because of its severe toxicity. Because of their toxicity and side effects, most of the DMARs and immunosuppressives used to treat human arthritis would be considered too dangerous for animals, especially having to monitor weekly blood tests. Except for vaccine preparations, the veterinarian's hands were tied until the safer and more effective tetracyclines and other antibiotics became available. One antibiotic, Tylosin, used by veterinarians for many years to successfully treat arthritis in animals, has not been approved for human use. Why not? New drugs usually are not introduced for approval unless profitable.

The kind of drugs or combination of drugs that are selected to provide maximum relief must be determined on an individual basis. The logic and choices behind current drug therapy have not been directed toward a suspected infectious viral-like agent. The selection of immunosuppressive drugs to control or cure an infectious disorder, especially viral, seems counterproductive with the loss or reduction of immune defenses against infections. Because of their more severe side effects, the immunosuppressants azathioprine and cyclophosphamide are usually prescribed after all other therapy has failed.

One might judge from the selection of new drugs for rheumatoid arthritis therapy that the clinical investigators were neither searching for a cure nor interested in finding the cause. Why should they when billions of dollars can be made from each new drug marketed? Rheumatoid arthritis has often been considered an autoimmune disorder related to the Graft-versus-host type of immunologic disorder, where a foreign organ or tissue transplant is rejected by the host. Several immunosuppressive drugs, including corticosteroids and cyclosporin, have been used to treat the so-called autoimmune diseases, where the host forms antibodies that react against its own tissues. In most cases, these autoimmune reactions are the immunologic results of the disease (rheumatoid arthritis, SLE, etc.) and not the primary cause but may still be responsible for additional symptoms.

Fearful Therapies
One of the latest and most infamous immunosuppressive drugs used for the treament of rheumatoid arthritis and other immunologic disorders is Thalidomide, the drug of birth defect fame. Used originally as a sedative, it was unfortunately prescribed to stop morning sickness in pregnant women and resulted in thousands of babies born in Europe (1959-1961) with malformed limbs. Thalidomide is now currently being used and investigated as a host-versus-Graft immunosuppressive in cancer patients receiving life-saving bone marrow transplants. A few doctors and researchers in other countries have reported that Thalidomide helps other immune system disorders, such as rheumatoid arthritis and SLE, in patients who do not respond to the usual therapy. Like the other immunosuppressive drugs prescribed for rheumatoid arthritis, Thalidomide could have other unknown dangerous side reactions while relieving symptoms. It makes one wonder whether Thalidomide could have some female predisposition, like many rheumatoid disorders. Why don't doctors try the less dangerous tetracyclines, which are also immunosuppressant and have sustained more than 40 years of safe and effective therapy?

FK 506
One of the newest and perhaps most effective and untested antirheumatic drugs is the Japanese manufactured immunosuppressant called FK 506, which is closely related to the macrolide antibiotic erythromycin. FK 506 is already being used successfully for organ transplants and the treatment of some autoimmune diseases,

such as psoriasis and kidney diseases. In test tube cell cultures, FK 506 is 10 to 100 times more immunosuppressive than its closest rival, cyclosporine, the current drug of choice for organ transplants. This new drug hopefully will be tested in some of the other major autoimmune disorders, such as rheumatoid arthritis, SLE, multiple sclerosis, diabetes, and Alzheimer's. Presently, the pharmaceutical manufacturer has limited its use, for some unknown reason, to organ transplantation. Of course if FK 506 is found to act like its related macrolide antibiotic, erythromycin, which inhibits mycoplasmas, it would greatly enhance its competitive and economic value in the world's health market.

Invasive Therapies

Perhaps the most extreme form of therapy that has been used in the more severe rheumatoid patients after all approved drugs have failed is a type of blood dialysis, similar to that used for kidney failure. One of the two most common forms is plasmaphoresis, where the blood cells are restored while the plasma is filtered to remove the suspected inflammatory agents, such as immune complexes. The other procedure removes a large portion of the surplus white blood cells which are suspected, as previously mentioned, as being the overactive cells causing the inflammatory and destructive enzyme action. The depletion of the white blood cells from the blood to control inflammation is comparable to removing hot charcoals from the grill in order to cool the fire. As one might suspect, the white blood cells depletion or irradiation (photophoresis) techniques do not remove the cause. Consequently, the very costly high-risk procedures are not readily accessible as the short period of benefit requires repetitive procedures.

Actually, these more recent invasive techniques are not any closer to a cure than those used 40 years ago when doctors had the patient's bad teeth and tonsils removed. They also advised splenectomies in the rheumatoid arthritis patients when some hidden bacterial foci was thought to be the cause. Why didn't some doctor put patients on high doses of antibiotics and thus avoid the painful and risky surgery? Fortunately, one doctor did pursue antibiotic therapy in preference to surgery. He hypothesized that some persistent, atypical infectious agent, such as mycoplasmas, may only respond to long-term rather than conventional short-term antibiotic therapy. Recently, synovectomies, another form of surgical treatment that removes the inflamed joint tissues, seem to have lost their popularity as the short-term benefits did not stop the course of the disease. Arthroscopic techniques, looking and probing into the joint spaces, although having some short-term therapeutic benefits, are primarily used for diagnostic purposes to detect and evaluate the extent of joint damage. When extensive damage is found associated with pain and immobility, orthopedic surgeons can repair and replace the damaged joint to restore function. Unfortunately, even this miraculous surgery does not remove the cause and thus is another form of palliative arthritis therapy.

Targeting the Infectious Causes

If investigators now suspect or believe that some persistent infectious agent is the cause of rheumatoid arthritis, why are they not testing every antibiotic on the shelf and then some? In the early 1930s, prior to antibiotics when gold was being used, investigators were looking for a bacterial cause of rheumatoid arthritis. As might be expected, many different strains of bacteria were isolated from the patient's throat, teeth, tonsils, stools, and other areas, and as many from the nonarthritis controls. At that time, some investigators believed that at least some arthritis cases were caused by a sensitized bacterial allergy. Arthritis symptoms were demonstrated when bacterial antigen (nonliving) was injected into a previously sensitized rabbit's knee joint. It is interesting to note that one of the Harvard Medical School investigators, Louis Dienes, was the first to isolate mycoplasma from humans (1934) and would later (1949) suggest the possible relation of human mycoplasma strains to articular disease. At that time, Brown reported the first successful use of tetracycline therapy in rheumatoid patients, especially after they had failed on the far more toxic gold therapy.

The Harvard investigators rightly rationalized that if rheumatoid arthritis was the delayed response to bacterial allergy, it might be possible to identify the culprit by skin testing, as they had done in tuberculosis. The patients were skin tested with several different strains of bacteria isolated directly from each patient. They found no significant difference in the skin tests with the bacterial vaccines between patients and controls, which thus did not allow the identification of any specific bacteria. They concluded that the skin test reactions did not support the hypothesis that rheumatoid arthritis is a disease of bacterial allergic origin.

About 50 years later, Clark and Brown conducted a similar investigation using six autologous strains of mycoplasmas for vaccine preparation and skin testing. Again, they theorized that if rheumatoid arthritis was caused by a mycoplasma hypersensitivity or a delayed allergic reaction, the patients should skin test positively to their autologous strain. In order to test this hypothesis, six different human mycoplasma strains were cultured with gamma globulin-free human sera to eliminate nonspecific reactions with the rheumatoid factor. The washed mycoplasma cells were suspended in saline to a constant protein concentration. Five micrograms of each vaccine preparation were injected in both forearms of 12 patients and asymptomatic controls. The patients' skin tests were usually more positive for their own autologous strain but also reacted to one or two other strains. When the mycoplasmas were also found to elicit delayed-type skin reactions in some of the asymptomatic controls, it became apparent that many people could first become sensitized to the deposited mycoplasmas, similar to subclinical Tb prior to expressing clinical systems. These observations indicated that inflammatory activity resulted from the subsequent exposure or release of cell-bound mycoplasma antigen into the sensitized host by physical or emotional stress. The rise in mycoplasma serum antibody titer induced following a drug-related Herxheimer's reaction or spontaneous stress flare is indicative of mycoplasma antigen release, like a booster shot. The persistence of both mycoplasma and its antibodies in the host indicates why mycoplasma vaccines are only partially effective in both animals and humans. The mycoplasma vaccines initiate neutralizing antibodies that are not very effective in removing the mycoplasmas and consequently are not an effective therapeutic modality. Our mycoplasma vaccine preparations were tested at monthly intervals in one rheumatoid arthritis patient, one asymptomatic control, and one rheumatoid gorilla. Both the patient and the gorilla improved, with a positive antibody response over a 6-month period. However, because the improvement did not hold, the vaccine boosters were

90

discontinued, not knowing what prolonged injections would introduce. In broader controlled studies, other investigators had reported that *Mycoplasma pneumoniae* vaccine in some subjects seemed to contribute to their pneumonia rather than protecting. Thus we learned again that mycoplasmas do not act or respond like bacteria and viruses even though they can also cause septic (infectious) arthritis usually of limited duration and unlike rheumatoid arthritis. It should be noted that many people can be infected with mycoplasmas without developing any noticeable clinical symptoms or disease. Our NIH grant application to pursue this research direction was not approved, and consequently the role of vaccines in controlling a potential infectious cause of rheumatoid arthritis has not been adequately pursued.

By now, researchers should realize and even predict that antibiotics will affect the membrane-bound (wall-less) mycoplasmas differently than the cell wall protected bacteria. Again, it seems necessary to ask why the safer antibiotics have not been tested in rheumatoid arthritis when some atypical infectious agent is the suspected cause. The atypical virus found to cause atypical pneumonia was atypical partly because, unlike most viruses, it was inhibited by tetracycline. Knowing that the small nonbacterial mycoplasmas were also inhibited by tetracycline, investigators tried and succeeded in showing both morphologically and metabolically that the atypical virus (Eaton agent) was actually another mycoplasma. As in animal models, tetracycline therapy had a minimal effect on the course of mycoplasma pneumonia unless given at the early onset. Even after therapy and symptoms abated, viable mycoplasmas were still shed and recovered from the patient's throats. Basically, tetracycline stops mycoplasma extracellular growth by inhibiting its ribosomal protein synthesis. Viruses require living cells to replicate their viral proteins and thus would be inhibited only by stopping the required cell growth, which tetracycline and other drugs could do in sufficiently high and toxic concentrations. If a viral cause of rheumatoid arthritis is expected, why not test antiviral drugs or vaccines?

A group of investigators who found that antiamoebic (antiparasite) drugs such as metronidazole or Flagyl benefited rheumatoid arthritis patients were led to believe that rheumatoid arthritis was caused by an amoebic infection. Why hasn't this approach been pursued and proven or disproven?

Taking Arthritis Treatment Seriously

When the National Arthritis Advisory Board (NAAB) reported to Congress in 1983 that the mycoplasma cause of arthritis should be taken seriously, why didn't they recommend a clinical trial of therapy with the safe and well-known tetracycline? Instead, they recommended the nearly impossible and costly task of first isolating or detecting mycoplasmas in the rheumatoid arthritis patient's synovial tissues prior to a clinical trial of tetracycline therapy. In sharp contrast, the Arthritis Foundation's *Primer of the Rheumatic Diseases* (1983) states that "despite numerous attempts to relate mycoplasma to RA, the accumulated evidence mitigates against such relationship." Furthermore, the primer listed tetracycline as a nonrheumatic drug even though tetracycline's effectiveness had never been adequately clinically tested for its antirheumatic activity. Why did the Arthritis Foundation tell doctors and patients that tetracycline is a nonrheumatic drug that does not help rheumatoid arthritis without having conducted the proper clinical trials that they had demanded from Brown?

Perhaps the NAAB experts considered it merely a coincidence that most of the recommended disease-modifying drugs (gold, hydroxychloroquine, copper-penicillamine, and even bee venom) are all antimycoplasma agents. When the so-called disease-modifying (DMAR) drugs become intolerable and ineffective, the next drugs of choice are the far more dangerous immunosuppressive drugs (cyclophosphamide, Azothioprine, cyclosporine) instead of testing the safer, multiple-action tetracyclines. The experts would have to agree that the demonstration of tetracycline's effectiveness in controlling rheumatoid arthritis, even with a concurrent decline in detectable mycoplasmas, would not prove their cause but only increase the supportive evidence for the hypothesis.

In 1981, the Arthritis Foundation's Unproven Remedies Subcommittee published a special article in the professional *Arthritis and Rheumatism* journal that stated: "A prominent Rheumatologist in the Mid-Atlantic area believes that he has proved that mycoplasmas cause arthritis and therefore treats RA patients with tetracycline, together with standard therapy. A prior controlled study in Boston ('71) denies this claim. He has chosen to promote his theories through the national media and his Institute rather than refereed journals and has expanded his claims to include gorillas and elephants with arthritis." If the committee had taken the time to check, they would have known that the prominent rheumatologist had published his claims and theories in medical text books, scientific journals, and even in their own *Arthritis and Rheumatism* journal as well as being accepted for presentation at international and national scientific rheumatology meetings. The Arthritis Foundation failed to recognize that Brown et al. were the first to report on the use of tetracycline for the treatment of rheumatoid disease in a refereed journal (J. Lab. Clin. Med. 34:1404-1410, 1949). They would also know that in the 1971 Boston study (Skinner et al.), tetracycline was included along with the standard toxic therapies and the prominent rheumatologist had opposed the use of the standard drugs (gold, antimalaria, penicillamine, and methotrexate) primarily because their severe toxicities are far greater than those of tetracycline. What would the average patients or doctors think when they saw this short note on unproven arthritis treatment interspersed with: Green-lipid mussel extract, Chuifong Toukiwan, Gerovital H3, Venoms, DMSO, Liefcort, etc.? When we asked one director at NIH why NIH did not test tetracycline, his answer was, "NIH can't support research on every laetrile [quack cancer remedy] that comes along." Ten years later, after patients demanded action, Congress requested NIH to conduct a clinical trial of tetracycline.

In an earlier article from *Aches & Pains*, distributed by Geigy Pharmaceuticals, entitled "Avoiding Quackery in Arthritis," it stated that "One physician who believes that mycoplasma causes arthritis has been treating patients with tetracycline. A controlled study failed to substantiate his claims, but the drug has still been promoted through the lay media, and its use has been extended to gorillas and elephants with arthritis. The humans who got the antibiotic received standard arthritis treatment simultaneously, which may explain their satisfaction with tetracycline treatment." This article, like the others, was also interspersed with references to venoms, vaccines, DMSO, and various hormones. Is this guilt by association? If that wasn't enough, the article further states that "The goal is not eradication of the disease but maintenance of function . . . . The patient should be encouraged to focus on living life normally with a tolerable level of pain and discouraged from focusing on a cure." If the Arthritis Foundation and the NIH goal is not the eradication of arthritis, whose goal is it? I am sure that the 40 million arthritic patients in America would like to know so that they can redirect their support.

Copper bracelets—Another View
The Arthritis Foundation has expressed the view that wearing a copper bracelet is a quack remedy for arthritis. However, a leading pharmacology professor believes that "not understood" would be a more accurate term than "quack." The copper bracelet has never been demonstrated to be ineffective against arthritis. A chemistry professor in Australia who had read of the pharmacologist's work on the anti-inflammatory action of copper aspirinate complex and related metal-binding chelates decided to scientifically test to see if the mythical value of copper bracelets might have a rational basis. Using noncopper control bracelets, he found chemical evidence that copper from the bracelets dissolves in sweat and enters the body through the skin, providing subjective evidence of therapeutic value against arthritis (see "Inflammatory Diseases and Copper," Ed J.R.J. Sorenson, Humana Press, 1982). Copper complexes were found to have anti-inflammatory activity. Copper enzymes play a role in tissue repair, and inflammation is made worse by copper deficiency. This evidence potentially could provide a better understanding of arthritis and hence better approaches to therapy. The evidence has gone unnoticed in part because of the connotation of quackery when copper is mentioned along with arthritis. Unfortunately, the state of the art of arthritis treatment has gone beyond the value of a copper bracelet, and such a study may not repay the costs when better sources of copper are available.

Establishing an unproven remedies list would include remedies that could be effective but remain untested or have been tested but failed to meet certain standards. They could provide 50-percent overall improvement to over one half the patients for a certain period. How a drug is tested or how the medicine is taken may also determine its benefits or harm. Thus ineffective (not beneficial) therapy for some patients may be effective for others. Because some drugs have multiple actions affecting multiple symptoms, the testing and evaluation of a drug's effectiveness should include the possible causative agents as well as the many resulting mechanisms and symptoms and over a longer period. One of the primary reasons there are so many hundreds of different forms of rheumatoid disorders is that patients symptomatically can respond differently to the same persistent irritant, especially if the infectious irritant targets and attaches to different tissues and in different amounts.

Until rheumatologists find a safe and effective treatment, desperate patients, when all approved therapies have failed them, will start searching and testing on their own to a tune of $2 billion a year. Many proposed therapies are now recognized as prohibitively costly, ineffective, and even dangerous. However, all new therapies that remain untested or whose claims are unsubstantiated should not be dumped automatically in the quackery barrel. Admittedly, some patients may have low serum copper levels and could benefit from copper therapy. The copper bracelet is comparable to the more modern transdermal patches except for the green copper oxide marking. The effectiveness is also dependent upon the amount and acidity of the patient's sweat. Who knows, perhaps some day the inventor or corporation that makes transdermal patches will prepare some with copper-tetracycline for rheumatoid skin disorders (psoriasis, scleroderma, etc.) New anti-inflammatory dermal lotions are continuously being proposed and tested and like so many other symptomatic band-aid therapies eventually fail by falling short of the cause.

Fact or Friction
In June 1981, a few months prior to the Arthritis Foundation's article on quackery, we had presented a paper entitled "Comparative Aspects of Rheumatoid Arthritis in the Gorilla and Man" at the XVth International Congress of Rheumatology in Paris. Because of the possible interest this report might have to the news media, we hired the same public relations firm used by the Arthritis Foundation (at a considerable expense) in order to get the facts straight in the news media. The public relations memo we released stated that:

"Gorillas help researchers provide new hope for arthritis sufferers. Great hope for sufferers from crippling arthritis through administration of appropriately spaced tetracycline, combined with anti-inflammatory agents, was held out here today by an internationally recognized rheumatologist.

"His principal partner in research is Tomoka, the 20-year-old star gorilla of the National Zoo in Washington, D.C. Dr. Brown told the Congress that Tomoka and twelve other gorillas in zoos worldwide have provided the basis for the conclusion that rheumatoid arthritis is a potentially curable and preventable disease. He identified it as caused by a unique group of virus-like microorganisms known as mycoplasmas. Dr. Brown, who reported on the comparative aspects of rheumatoid arthritis in the gorilla and man, based it on his 35 years of research on man and 12 years of parallel immunologic studies and treatment of gorillas.

"Mycoplasmas in both humans and gorillas were found to be identical and permitted demonstration that they have an affinity for joints and disease potential as a result of a severe allergic-type reaction. Dr. Brown and his associates have avoided studies with animal models with artifically-induced disease. Instead, they have directed their attention to the naturally occurring disease in a species closely related to man.

"Tomoka was first seen in 1969 at the request of the National Zoo in Washington, D.C. At that time he was scheduled for euthanasia because of severe crippling and painful arthritis. He had developed a resistance to all standard medications. Dr. Brown and his principal associate, Dr. Harold W. Clark, diagnosed Tomoka's problem as rheumatoid arthritis on the basis of clinical behavior and laboratory findings. They then started a treatment plan based on their previous success in the long-term management of human arthritis, utilizing the same principle and the same concept. (Having isolated a human mycoplasma strain and detected its antibody, I.V. tetracycline treatment was indicated.)

"A comparative 5-year follow-up of 35 humans with severe rheumatoid arthritis, similarly resistant to standard treatment methods, revealed a 70-percent average degree of improvement. A key to the program is the highly individualized spacing and dosage of the antibiotic, with concurrent anti-inflammatory agents, controlled

96

by the reactive state of the patient. This is unlike the standard treatment for infectious disease. The difference was that not until they were able to work with Tomoka were the researchers able to reinforce their concept with a controllable model stabilized in a constantly observable environment. While all previous medications, many of which are standard arthritis treatments today, had failed to arrest Tomoka's progressive disease, Dr. Brown reported, Tomoka's arthritis has now been in remission for 5 years and he shows no sign of disability. Similarly, 12 other gorillas in zoos around the world have responded favorably to the same treatment program.

"According to the study, mycoplasmas are specific for each animal species. The defense mechanism in man and gorilla is similar and highly sophisticated, and their host reactions create a different disease pattern than in lesser species. Rheumatoid arthritis is observed only in the higher species. Thus, while mycoplasmas are known to cause spontaneous arthritis in lower animals, it was not until the human strains of mycoplasmas were isolated from arthritic gorillas that a true spontaneous animal model was available.

"It was 83 years ago in 1898 at the Pasteur Institute in Paris that mycoplasmas (PPLO) were first isolated as the cause of arthritis in cattle. Thirty-two years ago (1949) at the 7th International Congress of Rheumatology we presented evidence for the causative role of mycoplasmas in the rheumatoid hypersensitivity mechanism. We noted the unique effect of tetracycline on the strains of mycoplasma isolated from arthritic patients and suggested a new therapeutic direction. The additional data presented today support the validity of this initial concept and provide the hope that through early definitive treatment the era of arthritis prevention will soon be at hand."

* * *

Whether it was the contents of the above memo or the action by the Arthritis Foundation's public relations firm or even the available copies of the report, the arthritis story made the front page of many newspapers and magazines around the world. Apparently the Arthritis Foundation was able to kill other pending stories and two days later issued the following "Public Information Memo 81-15" and a statement that was distributed to the chapter executive directors across the United States.

Dr. Thomas McPherson Brown/Gorillas/Mycoplasma/Tetracycline Therapy: Publicity and AF Statement:

You may be aware of newspaper and broadcast publicity in the last few days for an arthritis "cause-and-possible-cure" report attributed to a Dr. Thomas McPherson Brown and referring to studies of rheumatoid arthritis in gorillas.

The story was tied to a presentation by Dr. Brown during the International Congress of Rheumatology being held in Paris this week, but it was actually promoted via efforts of a PR firm in this country.

Attached is a statement by the Arthritis Foundation to help you in handling inquiries. It says in sum that despite his claims, neither Dr. Brown nor other researchers have actually proved that mycoplasma cause rheumatoid arthritis, nor is there valid evidence that tetracycline can cure the disease or even be of benefit to its victims.

The letter from the Vice President for Public Education stated:
"Dr. Brown is a prominent rheumatologist and has been associated with the Metropolitan Washington (D.C.) Chapter of the Arthritis Foundation. But the Foundation does not accept his claims about mycoplasma and tetracycline or condone high pressure publicity efforts made by Dr. Brown and his associates (notably Harold Clark, Director of Research at the Institute), to make their theories sound like actual break-throughs. Such publicity has been

aggressively sought for the past twelve years, and Dr. Brown has traveled and lectured enough to have stimulated formation of "Dr. Brown fan clubs" among patients in Alabama, Pennsylvania and elsewhere.

"We are unhappy that Dr. Brown still chooses to reject or bypass the accepted peer-review procedures of science, and to seek visibility for his theories and claims in a way that can only stir the hopes of arthritis sufferers without sufficient justification." The following statement was also attached to the above letter.

Arthritis Foundation Statement Concerning
Theory and Treatment of Thomas McPherson Brown, M.D.

"A medication therapy advocated by a Dr. Thomas McPherson Brown of Arlington, Virginia, is one of an apparently endless stream of methods proposed for the treatment of arthritis—without proper proof of effectiveness.

"It is Dr. Brown's theory that rheumatoid arthritis is caused by a specific organism called mycoplasma; and that it can be cured with antibiotics— specifically, tetracycline.

"For more than ten years, Dr. Brown has been citing studies involving gorillas to back up his claim. His idea is not at all new. Mycoplasma (a tiny form of life somewhere between bacteria and viruses) have been suspected as infectious agents in rheumatoid arthritis for many many years, have been the subject of much research, and have not been proved guilty. Dr. Brown himself has not provided scientifically valid evidence to support his theory. Neither have other researchers. So his idea remains a theory and only a theory.

"Because of this lack of proper medical evidence and proof obtained in clinical trials, the Arthritis Foundation classifies Dr. Brown's antibiotic therapy as an unproven remedy for arthritis, and does not recommend it.
In 1971, the scientific journal, Arthritis & Rheumatism, carried a report on a double-blind controlled trial of tetracycline in the treat-

ment of rheumatoid arthritis. It said the tests showed no benefit from tetracycline therapy.

"Further research on Dr. Brown's theory continues as just one part of overall research in which many other significant leads are being followed. Until such scientific studies provide reliable answers, we recommend that people with arthritis follow the established treatment procedures which have been proven effective in alleviating pain and preventing or reducing arthritis disabilities.

"The Foundation is very concerned about favorable publicity that has been given to Dr. Brown's ideas, and considers it premature and misleading. It is a disservice to arthritis sufferers whose hopes are raised by such reports."

Multiple Action Drugs Versus Shotgun Therapy

Many choices of symptomatic medications that are neither curative nor preventative are readily available by prescription or over the counter. Aspirin is one of the most diverse-acting medications, and it has been said that no other drug makes so many feel better. Salicylates, or aspirin, in their various forms have been used since Hippocrites (400 B.C.). As the father of medicine, he advised women to chew willow bark to relieve their pains of childbirth. Since the identification of their active ingredient (salicin) 200 years ago, salicylates have been concocted in many different forms—many claiming "arthritis strength" that relieves pain and many other symptoms. Although the nonsteroidal uses of aspirin continue to increase, the bases for its multifunctional actions are still relatively unknown. The rheumatoid arthritis patient's overloaded medicine cabinets and closets attest to the fact that not only is there no cure but the trial and error therapy with a multibarrel symptomatic approach has lost sight of any possible infectious cause or persistent irritant. Aspirin's multiple action depends on its complexed state, which could have negative or positive benefits. Even though aspirin remains the number one all-purpose medication, some of its mechanisms of action, such as boosting the immune system and preventing pregnancy complications, remain unexplained. As an anticoagulant complexing calcium, aspirin can improve blood flow to the eyes and thus benefit patients with diabetic retinopathy. This could also hold true for other chelating agents, such as vitamin C or even tetracyclines. When

100

chelated with copper, aspirins not only are more potent anti-inflammatory agents but also, as antioxidants (electron scavengers), could restrict cataract formation and even limit the damage caused by the chemical and radiation therapies for cancer. Yet shotgun therapy using multiple drugs is still in vogue trying to cover all bases or all symptoms.

Tetracyclines—Multiple Action Drugs

The broad range of rheumatoid diseases includes some of the most debilitating and costly diseases that we have had to endure. Primarily because of their baffling unknown causes and mechanisms, which can affect every tissue, therapy has been empirical and symptomatic and often with questionable long-term benefits.

Chelating Action: Intravenous Versus Oral Therapy

Whether mycoplasmas or other agents are the persistent sensitizing pathogens in rheumatoid diseases remains to be demonstrated. The primary concern is a safer and more effective alternative treatment to the toxic forms of therapy that impose a greater danger and economic burden. The tetracyclines are potent chelating (complexing) agents and as such have been found to act as anti-inflammatories, immunosuppressives, and antimetalloenzymes (anticollagenase), as well as antibiotics. When tetracyclines complex with copper, they become active antioxidants and anti-inflammatory agents. By complexing with the copper, zinc, iron, and other elements in the metalloenzymes, such as collagenase, tetracyclines can inhibit their destruction of the tissue-binding collagen protein. Consequently, the mode of tetracycline administration, intravenous or oral, could have a pronounced effect on their complexed state and thus their reactivity. The beneficial effects of tetracyclines or other chelating agents (aspirin, vitamins C, E, A, etc.) could be the results of their multiple actions, including antibiotic. For example, taking plain aspirin or vitamin C prior to tetracycline could tie up the available calcium and thus promote other more active forms of tetracycline, resulting in better absorption and utilization.

Bioassays for tetracycline levels in the blood and tissue fluids measure the antibacterial (antibiotic) activity but would not account for the other activities that are dependent upon its complexing

101

with trace metals and other tissue components. Consequently, the direct intravenous therapy into the blood stream would produce a more constant composition and activity than the highly variable, between meals, oral route even though the blood antibiotic activity levels were similar. Unlike other antibiotics, tetracyclines are prescribed between meals and especially not with high calcium milk and dairy products primarily because the calcium tetracycline complex is poorly absorbed in tissues.

Brown's original selection and use of tetracyclines as a safer alternative to the toxic gold therapy was based on the hypothesis that arthritogenic mycoplasmas, as in animals, may also be the cause of rheumatoid arthritis in humans. Finding that all rheumatoid patients did not respond equally to the same tetracycline dosage, Brown reported the first use of intravenous tetracycline to control severe rheumatoid arthritis and also the advantages of starting with small intermittent doses (Amer. J. Med. Sci., 221:618-624, 1951). In support of the successful treatment of humans and gorillas with rheumatoid arthritis, intravenous tetracycline treatment has also been reported to be more effective than oral doses in controlling mycoplasma arthritis in experimental mice.

Lyme disease, which resembles rheumatoid arthritis and rheumatic fever in its chronicity and difficulty to control and is caused by a spirochete from a tick-bite infection, has been found to be managed by intravenous tetracycline therapy. Like rheumatoid arthritis, the longer that Lyme disease persists the more difficult it is to control.

The beneficial effects of chelation therapy proposed by some investigators, including aspirin and ascorbic acid (vitamin C), is of special interest as ascorbic acid is often used to buffer tetracycline preparations for intravenous therapy. Another major factor to consider is tetracycline's cellular toxicity and primary function to inhibit protein synthesis, which is also dependent on its chelating activity. Tissue cells will survive intermittent (pulse) treatment of tetracyclines but not constant exposure even at lower doses. In rheumatoid arthritis, there apparently is no need to keep on top of a virulent infectious agent with high daily doses of antibiotics (as for bacteria). Instead, low dosage, intermittent therapy that is less toxic and less resistant seems to better control both the host's reactions and the foreign antigens.

What Is Proper Treatment?

A noted rheumatologist in London published an article on the "History of the Treatment of Rheumatoid Arthritis" in the British Medical Journal, 1:763-765, (1976) stating: "The treatment of an untreatable condition such as rheumatoid arthritis, calls forth great therapeutic skills and expertise. Anybody can cure a curable disease if they happen to have the right drug at hand, but the treatment of a condition for which there is no positive cure makes much greater demands on the doctor who has to be a practical pharmacologist, human being, psychiatrist, and father confessor—they have, in fact, to be a proper physician in the fullest sense of the word." When no certain cure exists and the physician does not make this extra effort, quack remedies tend to proliferate. Consequently, the history of cures is full of extraordinary forms of treatment for the various rheumatoid disorders. Rheumatoid sufferers live in high hopes that some day their doctor will find something effective, and for this reason, they are optimistic that any new form of treatment may be the cure. As a result, there is a long list of cures that seemed to work initially but are now strange and outdated.

As previously discussed, the influence of diet on the body's processes is very real and at the same time controversial, ranging from fasting to special diets. More recently, the association of arthritis with food allergies and the dietetic benefits of certain fatty acids from fish are being reconsidered for possible therapeutic directions. Statistics now indicate that the underweight and undernourished and not the overweight are at greater risk to develop arthritis. As in other disorders, the preclinical weight loss due to malabsorption or dietary deficiency may foreshadow some pending rheumatoid disorder. The fact remains that there are no simple answers or magic bullets for these complex questions. When some investigator offers a plausible new treatment theory, the critics and the establishment immediately pounce on it as not scientifically validated, and it thus remains an unsupported, untested, and unproven theory.

If the rheumatoid arthritis patients think they are confused about their disease and the possible causes and cures, they probably know a lot more about their disease, when, where, and how much it hurts and the effects of treatment, than do the expert specialists. In fact, many doctors would find it difficult if not impossible to provide a scientifically valid description of rheumatoid arthritis. As for treatment of these indescribable complex diseases over the past 50 years, one may read that what we are learning about arthritis treatment is potentially very exciting, but it is too early to translate these results into specific recommendations.

With so many failed cures at hand, it is not surprising that doctors have an agnostic and highly critical attitude, which is not always shared by the patients. Is the next new drug also going to fail? The danger here is that a useful drug may not be given by the skeptical doctor even though some patients may have gained real benefit. Like the early disbelief of other miracle treatments (penicillin and insulin) for many years by the medical profession, the untreated patients usually pay the price of professional incredulity or lack of real patient concern. Some may object that there is no real harm in inducing a placebo response as long as the drug is known to be safe and less toxic. There is no need to make unfulfilled promises that rheumatoid arthritis can cripple and disable unless checked by proper treatment. This implies that rheumatologists have a proven treatment that can stop the crippling and disabling effects of rheumatoid arthritis or claim that their proper treatment will control the disease and prevent deformities. These claims may apply to a few patients, while the vast majority continue down the road leading to wheelchairs and premature death as the approved disease-modifying drugs fail.

In searching for a safe and effective treatment of rheumatoid disorders, let's not throw the baby (tetracycline) out with the bath water (mycoplasmas). Tetracycline may be an effective cure, while mycoplasmas remain a suspected cause. Because of their unknown causes and origin, most chronic diseases have been or still are treated on a trial and error basis in an empirical fashion and aimed primarily at the elimination of symptoms, which are the result and not the cause of the disease. Many of the newer medications are refinements or improvements to enhance the benefits of an earlier drug used for other disorders, such as oral gold. Other new medications, such as tetracycline and the cancer drug

104

methotrexate, have been used to treat other diseases.

Gold salts were among the first antibiotics used to treat Tb and found to benefit rheumatoid arthritis patients and were later modified, making them less toxic and still effective. The modification of quinine, used in treating malaria (antimalarials), to chloroquine and hydroxychloroquine (Plaquenil) resulted in more effective treatment of some forms of arthritis, especially Lupus (SLE). But again like gold, the toxic side effects greatly curtailed its long-term use in most patients. When the adrenalcorticosteroids (cortisone) were first introduced as a miraculous cure for rheumatoid arthritis, it was short lived because of the pronounced side effects and even its morbidity associated with the initial high doses used. Later, other cortisone derivatives were synthesized in an effort to find more effective but less toxic compounds. Today, these steroids remain miracle drugs when used in controlled amounts and with close surveillance even though their mechanisms of action remain little known.

The Arthritis Foundation reported in 1976 that a cure for rheumatoid arthritis was not yet known but that effective treatment methods to control the disease and prevent deformities and crippling were known. If this sounds like double talk, perhaps it is, except for a few patients. Unfortunately, over the past few years, many of the so-called effective treatment methods using disease-modifying antirheumatic drugs (DMARDS) are now being recognized as having minimal or no effect on modifying the course and final outcome of the disease. Why some patients benefit from a drug and others do not may be related to the individual tolerance to that medication and the individual genetic susceptibility to the persistent causal agent. In any case, no approved drug used in treating rheumatoid arthritis actually stops the basic disease process by eliminating the causal agent. The prescribed drugs and some over the counter medications help reduce pain and inflammation or otherwise slow down and limit the symptoms and thus provide most patients some relief and restored activity. But for how long?

Most of the currently used medications are designated as nonsteroidal anti-inflammatory drugs (NSAIDS), indicating that they act like but are not the steroidal, cortisone-like drugs. These NSAIDS include salicylates, ibuprofens, indomethacins,

105

phenylbutazone, diclosenac, and many other variations, not to mention dozens more waiting to make their entrance. Then there are many more drugs that could be or should be considered as anti-inflammatory primarily because of their antioxidant activity, which is probably the greatest source of inflammation. The ability of vitamins C (ascorbic acid), A, and E to act as antioxidants and anti-inflammatories is now readily recognized and even being promoted in some circles. The recognition and acceptance of tetracycline antibiotics as multiacting antioxidants is finally being considered, and even being tested as antiarthritic drugs. Like many of the NSAIDS, tetracycline has been known since the 1950s to block the release or activation of the inflammatory and destructive lysozomal enzymes (collagenase) from the immunologically activated white blood cells. Why then has it taken 40 more years to be recognized and tested? Most drugs have been used empirically to treat rheumatoid arthritis not knowing why or how they acted. Some rheumatologists did not know that the gold salts and antimalarials they were prescribing for their rheumatoid arthritis patients could also inhibit mycoplasma growth.

The Mycoplasma Target

Rheumatoid arthritis is thought to be caused by some persistent infectious agent and has been referred to as an immune complex and autoimmune disorder. No agent or antigen has been implicated, however, except for the rheumatoid factor, an anti-antibody found in rheumatoid patients, which is the result of the disease and not the cause. The detection of the rheumatoid factor is diagnostic in many patients (80 percent) but does not correspond to disease activity. The activity could depend on the amount of tissue-fixed immune complex and not the discordant amount of immune complex in the blood circulation. In a 1988 study, Clark et al. found mycoplasma antigens in the immune complex isolated from the blood and joint fluid from rheumatoid arthritis patients. They also found that the mycoplasma cells complexed with serum immune globulin (IgG) caused the production of the anti-IgG (autoimmune) rheumatoid factor activity in rabbits but not arthritis. This is the first study that indicates the potential role of mycoplasmas in both the autoimmune and immune complex mechanisms seen in rheu-

106

matoid disorders.

In 1993, the U.S. Senate requested NIH to initiate intravenous tetracycline clinical trials, which should also monitor the mycoplasma antibody levels present in rheumatoid patients. Antibody levels were first reported by our research laboratory in 1964. Since then, our laboratory has tested thousands of patients' sera for antibodies to several human strains of mycoplasmas. These tests are still not available in other laboratories. The mycoplasma complement fixation test (MCF), which reflects mycoplasma infections, is not a diagnostic test for rheumatoid diseases. However, the MCF test has been used by doctors as a serologic yardstick to evaluate the response to antibiotic therapy and any associative changes, such as Herxheimer's flare, blood chemistry, hematology, and other clinical responses. Mycoplasmas are ubiquitous agents with frequent isolations from the genitourinary tract. Positive mycoplasma antibodies were found in many patients (80 percent) at infectious disease and venereal disease clinics. Of special interest was the observation that the incidence of mycoplasma antibodies in the female patients was four times that in the males, which coincidentally is approximately the incidence ratio found in rheumatoid arthritis patients.

There is no question that mycoplasmas can cause arthritis in humans. Whether they also cause the more persistent and progressive rheumatoid diseases remains the big question. If so, how should they be treated? Once the disease progresses and becomes chronic, the mycoplasmas apparently become firmly attached to the tissues and are thus very difficult to isolate and treat. As some strains of mycoplasmas are currently recognized as pathogenic agents (*M.pneumoniae, M.hominis*), positive antibody production to these or other strains, especially after initiating tetracycline therapy, would provide further justification for tetracycline (not penicillin) therapy. Mycoplasmas can continue to persist even after routine tetracycline therapy. The problem is that tetracyclines are immunosuppressive agents as well as inhibitors of protein synthesis and thus could also restrict the antibody production and detection. For this and many other conditions, a negative mycoplasma antibody test does not prove their absence.

Like other inflammatory diseases, the rheumatoid diseases

are apparently initiated by immune complexes or altered tissue antigens attached to specific cell receptor sites and thus not infectious and transmissible in the conventional sense. Consequently, investigators should not expect to find the usual high antibody titers found in infectious diseases. Over the past 10 years, the multiple effects of tetracyclines have been well documented. Their anti-inflammatory and immunosuppressive action could help to keep rheumatoid diseases under control without being antagonistic. The more vascular tissues and organs are more likely to be targeted, hence the term collagen vascular disorders, indicating the destruction of the collagen protein in blood vessels and other tissues. Tests of the rheumatoid arthritis patient's joint fluid for mycoplasmal antibodies and rheumatoid factor are frequently positive prior to their blood tests, indicating an initially localized joint tissue response. Even though viable mycoplasmas are infrequently isolated in the presence of mycoplasma antibody, the administration of localized intra-articular antimycoplasma therapy should also be considered.

Tetracyclines for Juvenile Rheumatoid Arthritis?
A potential solution for treating Juvenile Rheumatoid Arthritis, has been seriously overlooked or avoided. Like rheumatoid arthritis, the cause of Juvenile Rheumatoid Arthritis remains unknown, with girls being affected twice as often as boys. Aspirin and NSAIDS continue to be the drugs of first choice, with the more dangerous and toxic steroids, gold, antimalarials, and penicillamine close in line. The major hazards facing the 250,000 juveniles with rheumatoid arthritis include cardiac failure, deforming polyarthritis, and blindness in addition to the dangerous therapy that can appreciably increase their mortality rate. Because of their age (under 18 years), most clinical trials of NSAIDS and the more toxic DMARS excluded juveniles, making therapeutic selection experimental with questionable procedural risks.

Again, the big question is why pediatricians have not used the much safer tetracycline antibiotics in juveniles, especially when mycoplasmas or some other atypical infectious agent was suspected to be a cause of rheumatoid arthritis in adults. Our clinic and a few other doctors found tetracycline therapy to be highly effective with minimal side effects. A doctor in Hartford first reported in 1954

108

using tetracycline (Aureomycin) for known growth delay in avascular necrosis of the femoral epiphysis or hip deformities (LCP syndrome). He found that a small daily supplement of 50 mg of tetracycline hastened the regeneration of the upper femur. In a 1965 study, the doctor reported a double-blind trial of 54 children with hip disease (LCP syndrome). A 50 mg capsule of tetracycline, plus vitamins and minerals, or a placebo without tetracycline was given daily with breakfast. After 30 to 74 months, the tetracycline was found to hasten reossification and restoration of the femur and acetabulum (leg and hip) in 97 percent of the children as well as favorable influence on structural growth in 76 percent with no complications. Exactly what additional role the vitamin and mineral supplement played in this long-term oral tetracycline therapy remains speculative. Like the safe and effective long-term use of tetracycline therapy in juvenile acne, the question remains why tetracycline therapy has not been clinically tested in Juvenile Rheumatoid Arthritis by many more doctors. This question was recently answered by the front page headlines reporting that a researcher had found that an acne drug soothed rheumatoid arthritis when tetracycline was found to significantly reduce symptoms.

Being smaller and not fully developed, juveniles would be expected to react differently to the same etiologic mechanism and cause of adult rheumatoid arthritis. The symptoms in juveniles may be different but not the therapy. Variations in symptoms do not necessarily indicate different causes and different treatment unless, like most, the treatment is directed toward the symptoms and not the cause.

Therapeutic Inhibition of Collagen Diseases

Many of the enzymes that control oxidative metabolism (respiration), protein synthesis, and other biochemical functions are complexed with certain trace metals, such as iron, copper, zinc, manganese, and magnesium. All of these enzymes have very specific and essential life-sustaining functions. Some of these enzymes may lay dormant until activated by some challenge such as a foreign substance. For example, when food enters the stomach and intestines, active enzymes are released that hydrolyze or digest the food without digesting the stomach tissues, except under special conditions that promote gastric inflammation, resulting in ulcerative tissue destruction.

Perhaps one of the most damaging digestive metalloenzymes that is activated by inflammation is called collagenase because it digests the collagen protein that cements or holds the tissue cells together. Collagen is one of the major structural proteins of cartilage, skin, bone, blood vessels, and almost every tissue. The so-called collagen vascular disorders include most of the rheumatic diseases, where the collagen of the blood vessels is destroyed. Connective tissue disorders have the collagen in the connective joint tissues destroyed. The enzyme collagenase is stored primarily in the white cell granules. When an irritant such as an infectious agent or its immune complex attaches to tissue cells, white cells from the blood supply are attracted to the site, releasing their granules (lysozomes) of digestive collagenase and other enzymes. This is the body's key defense mechanism that destroys infectious agents or other irritants. The only problem is that if the condition persists, as in rheumatoid arthritis, excessive collagenase and other proteolytic enzymes are released from the over-abundant supply of localized white blood cells, resulting in the destruction of surrounding tissues. Thus three palliative solutions are presented: (1) remove the surplus white blood cells by physical and chemical means, (2) chemically inhibit the release or activation of the lysozomal enzymes, or (3) chemically inhibit the collagenase and other enzymes. These actions could still leave the persistent irritant and not stop the disease. Most of the NSAIDS used in treating arthritis, including tetracyclines, limit or reduce the release of the activated lysozomal enzymes.

Collagenase was identified in 1967 in the inflamed synovial tissues from rheumatoid arthritis patients and in the white cell granules associated with periodontal disease. It wasn't until 1982, however, that a group of dentists trying to explain the breakdown of oral collagen in connective tissues associated with diabetes found that collagenase was inhibited by tetracyclines. Tetracyclines, known strictly for their antimicrobial activity, had been used successfully for the treatment of various periodontal disorders. At first, because of their antibiotic properties, such disorders that also developed diabetes were believed to be caused by some gram-negative microorganism. Further studies showed that tetracyclines, but not the non-tetracycline antibiotics, reduced collagenase activity in both conventional diabetic rats and germ-free diabetic animals. The investigators concluded that this special therapeutic property, anticollagenolytic, of tetracyclines could be successfully used in treating diseases that involve excessive collagen destruction such as the collagen vascular disorders, including rheumatoid arthritis. These investigators reached the same prediction of tetracycline's effectiveness that Brown had 30 years before, only for different reasons, which was to eliminate the cause and not just the results of the disease.

The multiple nonantibiotic activities of tetracyclines were further recognized when it was apparent that the calcium and zinc metal ions in the collagenase enzyme were bound by the chelating tetracycline, thus inhibiting the collagenase activity. This was further supported by the inhibition of mammalian collagenase activity by a chemically modified nonantibacterial tetracycline. Almost like the story of insulin in treating diabetics, Brown, for over 40 years (1948-1988), had been successfully treating his rheumatoid patients with connective (collagen) tissue disorders using tetracyclines believing its action was primarily antimycoplasmal. In fact, he believed that all connective tissue diseases can be treated equally. One doctor in Washington, D.C., who realized that there was a similar mechanism involved, successfully treated some of his diabetic retinopathy and gangrene patients with tetracycline therapy until the medical society threatened to withdraw his medical license.

Diabetes, rheumatoid arthritis, and other disorders (SLE, Multiple sclerosis, Alzheimer's) all seem to have an autoimmune mechanism activity associated with or attributed to some unknown infectious agents. Even though they may each have a different or even the same mycoplasma cause, their beneficial and effective control by tetracycline treatment could be the result of tetracycline's anti-inflammatory, antioxidant, antimetabolite, and immunosuppressive activities and not just antibiotic. In a 1985 study, the dental investigators found that the oral administration of 100 mg of minocycline twice a day for 10 days significantly decreased (67 percent) the collagenase activity in the synovial tissue and fluid from seven rheumatoid arthritis patients. Each patient served as the before and after controls as in Brown's studies. When and how oral tetracycline was taken was not discussed but could explain the different levels and variable collagenase inactivation achieved.

Apparently referring to our studies, the authors indicated that "For many years an unconventional approach has advocated tetracycline antibiotics for the treatment of RA— despite the fact that the evidence in support of such therapy is entirely anecdotal and uncontrolled. The rationale for this approach (the hypothesis that RA has a mycoplasmal etiology) remains conjectural at best and that data in support of this treatment has appeared only in non-peer reviewed forums." What these authors failed to mention was that this so-called unconventional tetracycline approach, which they also confirmed and recommended, benefitted their rheumatoid arthritis patients as well as decreased collagenase activity. By confirming our results, I would hardly call them anecdotal or conjectural.

It is indeed tragic, at least for the millions of arthritic patients, that investigators, believing that some unknown infectious agent is the cause, continue to seek drugs tht only modulate the consequences or resulting symptoms of rheumatoid diseases and not a suspected infectious agent. Could not the tetracycline antibiotics be inhibiting both the infectious cause and destructive collagenase activity? In the meantime, the experts are advising that most people with arthritis should learn to live with the disease and that arthritis is a signal telling them that their bodies need more exercise.

Fortunately, many doctors are no longer waiting for the compelling evidence but for some reason are now treating their rheumatoid patients with tetracyclines either as an anticollagenase, anti-inflammatory, antioxidant, immunosuppressant, antibacterial, or antimycoplasma therapy. A group of doctors in the Netherlands recently reported on their open clinical trial of oral minocycline in 10 rheumatoid arthritis patients, supplementing the standard therapy with increasing amounts up to 400 mg/day for 16 weeks. The tetracycline-treated patients improved significantly over their pretreatment values, leaving the investigators to conclude that minocycline may be beneficial in rheumatoid arthritis but a much larger controlled trial is warranted. They have now conducted a long-term controlled trial in over 100 patients. The results of this successful study were reported at the Second International Symposium on the Immunotherapy of the Rheumatic Diseases in 1993. Unfortunately, many of these investigators, who recently have started their rheumatoid patients on tetracycline therapy, have failed to recognize or acknowledge that Brown and our research team pioneered and developed the tetracycline approach.

Investigators in Israel testing minocycline in 18 rheumatoid arthritis patients concluded:

"Our open trial suggests a beneficial effect of minocycline in patients with resistant RA who failed on two or more DMAR drugs. If this is confirmed in future controlled trials then minocycline may offer an attractive alternative therapy for RA, since its known side effects are not severe and subside after discontinuation of therapy." Unfortunately, this study was also published without any search or measure of an infectious etiologic agent or any reference to Brown's extensive pioneering efforts in first reporting (1949) the successful use of tetracycline in rheumatoid arthritis patients.

The recent confirmation of minocycline's effectiveness by the NIH multicenter trial MIRA, published in the Annals of Internal Medicine (1/15/95), finally recognized tetracycline as another therapeutic choice for rheumatoid arthritis and other rheumatoid diseases.

As the interest and acceptance of tetracycline therapy increases, we can only hope that the doctors do not repeat the earlier failures by using excessive doses of tetracyclines as just another antibacterial agent in an infectious disease. In time, they will learn and explore, as we did, the many problems and pitfalls encountered in a totally new world of the pharmacological basis of therapeutics that even the double-blind trials fail to solve. Now, in times of economic crisis and the urgent need to revise the nation's total health care program, the patients must step forward and call the shots, telling the medical providers and researchers what is delinquent and what is missing!

Chapter VII
The Case For Antimycoplasma therapy

In 1972, both the House of representatives and the Senate reported, in their appropriations for the National Institutes of Health (NIH), the need to investigate mycoplasmas as a cause of rheumatoid arthritis. The House reported: "Heartening progress is being made in determining the cause of rheumatoid arthritis. Recent research indicates that arthritis may be due to a so-called autoimmune reaction in which the body over-reacts to proteins originating with its own tissues. This reaction may be triggered by initial changes brought about by an infectious process. Institute scientists have produced in pigs a form of arthritis, resembling the human disease, by injecting the animals with certain mycoplasma organisms. The data obtained provided significant evidence of eventual and continued local antibody production in the joints even after the acute infectious process had run its course. The Institute (NIH) is pursuing this line of research, together with efforts to find new and improved agents for the management of all forms of arthritis." Note that there was no mention of veterinarians already using antimycoplasma therapy, such as tetracyclines, to eliminate the suspected mycoplasma cause of the pig's arthritis.

The Senate reported: "The search for causes of the main, crippling form of arthritis, rheumatoid arthritis, seems to have narrowed to a disorder of immune mechanisms possibly triggered by an initial infectious process. Pigs which develop a form of joint involvement resembling human rheumatoid arthritis, after injection with mycoplasma organisms, are providing information that may lead to clarifying the precise errors in immune response. The joints of these animals continue a type of 'immunochemical warfare' (*continued mycoplasma antibody production*) even after the acute mycoplasma infection has subsided." Again, these reports are summaries of earlier research presented by NIH to justify its continued and increased annual appropriations, which may or may not be used to support research grants in that area.

Unique Properties of Mycoplasma

Ten years later (1982), Clark et al. summarized the case for the mycoplasma cause of rheumatoid arthritis citing at least 12 properties supporting the role of mycoplasmas in rheumatoid arthritis. This summary was reported at the International organization for Mycoplasmology meeting and published in the Reviews of Infectious Diseases, Vol. 4, 1982. A number of unique properties of mycoplasmas support the role of these organisms as etiologic agents in rheumatoid arthritis: (1) Mycoplasmas are recognized as arthritogenic and systemic causative agents in several domestic animals, with apparent strain and species specificity. (2) Colonization (infection) of both the nasopharyngeal and genitourinary tracts by mycoplasmas is a common occurrence, affecting four times as many women as men, a predilection that would be a prerequisite to assigning these organisms a role in prevalent rheumatoid arthritis, which predominantly affects women (4:1). (3) Several strains isolated from the same or different animal species have marked physical and chemical variations. The pleomorphic characteristic of these organisms (the result of the lack of a cell wall), which also have unusual growth cycles and growth requirements, contributes to the difficult problem of mycoplasma identification in host tissues. (4) The low cytotoxicity of some strains of mycoplasma that had gone undetected in tissue cell cultures by the virologists would also support the finding of a low-titer antibody response and the persistence of these organisms even in asymptomatic hosts. (5) The finding that the greatest incidence of mycoplasmal antibodies in humans is associated with other infections would indicate that some mycoplasma strains are

116

commensal or secondary invaders, as recently reported to be associated with HIV infection in AIDS patients. (6) Mycoplasmas are difficult to eliminate from their infected host with antibiotics, or vaccines, a factor that indicates mycoplasmas persist fixed in or on tissues; such persistence could account for the infrequency with which the organisms are isolated from rheumatoid arthritis tissues. (7) The observed rise in antibody titer to specific mycoplasmas and a delayed-type inflammatory response following trauma or antimycoplasma therapy indicate the release of a persistent antigen (Herxheimer's reaction). (8) The well-known characteristic of mycoplasmas, i.e., that their composition mimics their growth media, would contribute to the production of autoimmune antigens, especially when the proteins assimilated during growth induce tissue-specific responses. Some strains of mycoplasmas are known to cross-react with different tissues such as brain, heart, and lungs. (9) Localized and persisting mycoplasma antibodies are frequently found in the synovial joint fluid and blood of patients with rheumatoid arthritis. The titer of mycoplasma antibodies in the blood frequently are inversely correlated with the titer of rheumatoid factor (anti-antibody). (10) Mycoplasmas participate in several cell-mediated responses, particularly the immunologic reactions of the delayed-type skin test. (11) The immunosuppressive effect of mycoplasmas on the reactivity of peripheral T lymphocytes or white blood cells is comparable to the suppressor activity associated with autoimmune responses. (12) The variety of substances empirically used to treat rheumatoid arthritis patients (antimalarial drugs, gold or copper salts, bee venom, penicillamine, and tetracycline antibiotics) also inhibit mycoplasmal growth. These various medications also can produce an inflammatory Jarisch-Herxheimer reaction, with a resulting rise in the mycoplasmal antibody titer.

Since that report, several more mycoplasma properties supporting their role in rheumatoid arthritis have been identified and will be discussed later.

Examination of Mycoplasma and Antimycoplasma therapy

The House Appropriations Committee in 1983 reported (H.R. 7205) that research has demonstrated that infectious agents and defects in the body's immune system are implicated in some types

117

of arthritis, a disease that affects over 31 million Americans. In preliminary studies total body lymphoid irradiation was shown to improve rheumatoid arthritis in some patients unresponsive to conventional therapies. "The committee has been approached by persuasive advocates for the antimycoplasma approach to the treatment of rheumatoid arthritis. The committee requests that the Institute (NIH) make a careful examination of the state of the art of this approach and report to it on the basic research undertaken and presently underway on this method of treatment."

In response to this request, the Deputy Director of NIH submitted a report to the House entitled "Mycoplasmas and Antimycoplasmal Treatment: A Review of Their Role in Rheumatoid Arthritis," which was published in the House hearings for 1984, Part 9. The report concluded that: "While one can not absolutely dismiss the hypothesis that mycoplasmas have a role in rheumatoid arthritis, the weight of current evidence is heavily against that possibility and does not warrant the initiation of a long term, multi-center clinical trial of tetracycline treatment of rheumatoid arthritis." The question remains, why would NIH want to dismiss the hypothesis before it has been tested, especially when they have no other effective therapy?

This NIH report preceded the May 1983 testimony of Brown requesting the funding of mycoplasma clinical research toward the cause and treatment of arthritis. Upon receiving a copy of the NIH report to the House committee, it was thoroughly examined and found to be inaccurate, containing many prejudicial omissions, and essentially nonresponsive to the committee's specific request. Because of the possible detrimental affects from the negative NIH report, Clark and Brown prepared and submitted a rebuttal statement on "The Antimycoplasma Approach to the Treatment of Rheumatoid Arthritis" in May 1983, which was also published in the House hearings for 1984, Part 9, 714-741. A copy of this report follows.

118

Mycoplasmas
80,000 x magnification

119

THE ARTHRITIS INSTITUTE
of the National Hospital, Arlington, Virginia
Statement on
The Antimycoplasma Approach to the
Treatment of Rheumatoid Arthritis

In Response to the Report

by the National Institutes of Health
of the Department of Health and Human Services
(February 1983)

Harold W. Clark, Ph.D.
Director of Research

Thomas McP. Brown, M.D.
Director
May, 1983

120

Introductory Statement

The Committee on Appropriations requested in House Report No. 97-894 that the Institute (NIADDK), as part of the FY 1983 budget (HR7205) make a careful examination of the state of the art of the antimycoplasma approach to the treatment of rheumatoid arthritis (RA) and report to the committee on the basic research undertaken and presently underway on this method of treatment.

In response to this request Thomas E. Malone, Deputy Director of NIH, submitted a 21 page report dated February 1983 entitled "Mycoplasmas and antimycoplasmal treatment: A review of their role in rheumatoid arthritis."

The review included three major areas of research on mycoplasmas: (1) detection, (2) immune response, and (3) treatment, concluding that: the weight of current evidence is heavily against the possibility that mycoplasmas have a role in rheumatoid arthritis and advised against a clinical trial of tetracycline treatment of rheumatoid arthritis at this time but stated that "research with mycoplasma-induced arthritis in animals, a useful model of arthritis, is continuing."

The Arthritis Institute of the National Hospital in Arlington, VA, as one of the foremost mycoplasma centers and the most experienced in clinical trials of antibiotic treatment of rheumatoid arthritis has reviewed the NIH report in detail and found it to contain inaccuracies and to be only partially responsive to the specific information requested by the House and Senate Appropriations Committees.

The weight of evidence that justifies continued support of animal research on mycoplasma-induced arthritis should also justify its application to the human disease, especially clinical trials on rheumatoid arthritis patients with safer and less costly drugs found effective in the arthritic animal models.

Weighing the Evidence:

1. While it is true that the detection or isolation of mycoplasmas (or any microorganism) from rheumatoid arthritis patients have been infrequent, this is also the case in experimental animals with mycoplasma induced arthritis where the mycoplasmas became non-recoverable (1). Hence, in view of the "useful" animal mod-

121

els the basis for requiring mycoplasma isolation from all patients is not a valid one. Note: Recently improved isolation techniques (E. Jansson, 1983) revealed the presence of mycoplasmas in rheumatoid arthritis patients' joint fluids.

2. The identification of mycoplasma antibodies in rheumatoid arthritis patients' blood has not been all positive. It is well known that the presence of blood antibodies are not essential for the occurrence of rheumatoid arthritis, Also the presence of anti-antibodies (rheumatoid factor) in the blood of rheumatoid arthritis patients (80%) reduces the potential for detecting mycoplasmas antibody levels. Thus the inability to detect antibodies in all rheumatoid arthritis patients should not be considered as negative evidence for antimycoplasma clinical trials (Clark, et al., 1976).

3. The NIH report based the ineffectiveness of tetracycline in treating rheumatoid arthritis patients on the results of a study obtained 12 years ago from one small and inadequate trial of a few patients on low oral dosage in combination with steroids and other drugs. Subsequent studies on arthritic animals showed that injectable and NOT oral tetracycline therapy was essential for the control of mycoplasma-induced arthritis in animals (4, 5, 8).

In view of the toxicity potential of gold salts and other approved drug therapies and their resultant high costs, the successful control of animal arthritis would surely warrant similar clinical trials with appropriate injectable dosages of the safer and more effective antibiotics (gold salts are also injectable doses). Such clinical trials of injectable and individualized dosages are especially warranted in humans because of earlier history of the limited effectiveness of oral tetracycline in controlling the late phase of *Mycoplasma pneumoniae* infections. Also the effective long term control of rheumatoid arthritis in several gorillas (closest animal model to humans) by veterinarians using this method further supports this position (6).

In a recent review of Mycoplasmas as arthritogenic agents two prominent investigators (Cole and Ward, 1979) supported for over 20 years by NIH grants and contracts concluded that "Mycoplasma induced arthritis (in animals) does not in general respond well to the usual doses of antibiotics but that continually applied high doses may exhibit a beneficial effect" (37).

122

Although they did not refer to any clinical trial on rheumatoid arthritis patients their conclusions certainly support the inadequacy of low oral doses and the need for a long term clinical trial with high antibiotic doses.

In the 1920's a French doctor (Forestier) testing the effect of gold salts on tuberculosis noted that those patients with rheumatoid arthritis responded to the treatment (32). Having found gold to help the patients' arthritis but not their TB, other doctors have continued to use the toxic and costly gold treatment empirically over the past 60 years (13).

Another physician (Thomas McP. Brown) noted, as did Dr. Albert Sabin, that gold was specifically effective against mycoplasmas (33), and further found that a far less toxic substance, tetracycline, was even more effective than gold in treating arthritis (38). After 35 years of extensive clinical and basic investigations, involving thousands of arthritic patients (and 18 arthritic gorillas), Dr. Brown has published additional information which heavily supports the use of antibiotics as a much safer, less costly, and more effective treatment and thus permits readily accessible and sustained long term treatment not possible with gold (7).

Until the infectious causes of rheumatoid arthritis are known, the real issue to be examined is what approach to the treatment of rheumatoid arthritis offers the greatest benefits at the lowest risk and cost. Rather than continue blindly with the empirical and symptomatic approaches to treatment fraught with dangerous side effects and limitations of usefulness, a basic mechanistic approach directed towards a treatable microbial antecedent offers not only therapeutic advantage but enlarged understanding. If Dr. Forestier was weighing the current evidence today he certainly would not select gold salts as the drug of first choice. Gold has been reported to be the most toxic drug in the Pharmacopeia and for one period was associated with the highest mortality rate (Gumpel, 1978).

Quite unlike acute infectious diseases, rheumatoid arthritis is not a simple problem related to joint inflammation but a progressive systemic disorder, with many different variations that can affect every tissue in the human host. Short term drug trials using double blind controls are appropriate for infectious diseases of limited duration and variable but not for slow acting microorganisms and chronic diseases affecting multiple tissue systems with multiple host responses. Double blind controlled studies are only "statistical short cuts" that attempt to determine in a very short time frame and with only a few patients what will apply over a long period to the total patient population. The many variations of the disease patterns in individual rheumatoid patients, the complex nature of the disease mechanism, and the long period usually required to bring the disease under control make a protracted double blind study completely uncontrollable and unreliable. This is evident by the many drug failures found even after short term double blind trials. It is known that rheumatoid patients develop delayed reactions to drugs that have appeared after the short trial has ended (21).

The 1971 controlled study cited in the NIH report as demonstrating no significant benefit to rheumatoid arthritis patients from tetracycline was far from controlled by a small group of 13 patients treated for only one year (39). Although some of the treated patients were found to benefit, they could not be reported as significant because of the small sample. Because of the small number of rheumatoid arthritis patients selected, the random distribution of medication produced two significantly different groups as to sex ratio, duration of illness, and concurrent medications which are all critical factors. Consequently the results obtained from this study comparing two unrelated groups (like oranges and apples) invalidate any conclusions.

For example:

The male:female incidence ratio in rheumatoid arthritis patients is usually 1:4 or .25. The reported study compared a .62 male:female group ratio with a .12 group ratio which are markedly dissimilar having a significant five-fold difference. Studies have shown that the eradication of mycoplasmas was more difficult in females requiring longer and higher doses of antibiotics.

Although the prior duration of rheumatoid arthritis has been found to significantly influence the response to treatment, the reported study compared one group with an average five years duration and the other with 9.5 years (a significant two-fold difference).

Although anemia and nodules are characteristic symptoms

124

in rheumatoid arthritis, the reported study had five times as many anemic patients and twice as many with nodules in one group.

When two groups are significantly different in the critical areas the whole basis for a control group would be negated and any comparison invalid. Fortunately the 1971 study did not show a significant improvement in the treated group. Otherwise it would have given the *false* impression that low dosage oral tetracycline would benefit all rheumatoid arthritis patients within a one year period.

For NIH to accept and support this short term, pseudo-controlled study of 13 inadequately treated rheumatoid arthritis patients in preference to a successful long-term trial on 35 patients as the basis for treatment indicates a much greater need for a thorough investigation of the evaluation process of other clinical trials. Withholding a safer, less costly, and highly rational clinical trial from the millions of arthritic patients solely on the basis of the unknown etiology of rheumatoid arthritis and the failure of one nonsignificant clinical trial to confirm antibiotic usage is wholly unjustified and should be seriously questioned by the medical community and the public if left unchallenged. Continuing to use more dangerous and costly drugs on an empirical basis while refusing to try safer and less costly antibiotics on a very rational basis until the cause is proven is totally incongruous (16-24).

When the lives of 35,000,000 arthritics are hanging in the balance at a cost of nearly $30,000,000,000/yr and increasing rapidly, the Federal Government cannot afford to overlook any possible cause and solution that offers promise.

Additional Evidence:
In searching for the best approach to treatment it is not enough to consider only the etiologic agent(s) and its effect on the host but should also include the host's responses to the microorganism. (The host's immune response can be more damaging than the infectious agent.) Thus, in considering whether gold salts, antimalarials (chloroquines) or tetracycline should be used to treat rheumatoid arthritis the doctors should be well aware that these drugs also have many properties in common such as: antibacterial, anti-inflammatory, immunosuppressing, antimetabolic, etc., including their

125

antimycoplasma activity (16).

The author(s) of the NIH report apparently were either unfamiliar with mycoplasmas and the treatment of rheumatoid arthritis or chose to avoid discussing and citing key references. As indicated on page 4, the author(s) did not know that the origin of mycoplasma or pleuropneumonia-like organisms (PPLO) dates back to 1898—their first isolation from cattle with pleural pneumonia (9). Neither did the author(s) seem to know (or failed to discuss) that antimalarials and other drugs used in the treatment of rheumatoid arthritis are also antimycoplasma agents (10), a very significant fact.

The author(s) of the NIH report stated (page 9) that (since 1971), "No further clinical trials of antimycoplasma treatment of humans with rheumatoid arthritis have been reported." This is an incorrect statement as the director of NIH was familiar with a report published by Brown et al. in 1982 (7) on a five year study of 35 severe rheumatoid arthritis patients and referred to this clinical trial in a letter (January 1983) to Senator Robert Byrd. Both the associate director for arthritis and the director of NIADDK had been given copies of the 1982 publication. Even the medical director of the Arthritis Foundation had received a copy of the 1982 publication and had personally discussed it with Dr. Brown.

Prior to the 1982 publication, a brief report on the antimycoplasma treatment program had been given at the XVth International Congress of Rheumatology in 1981. This report was published in the abstracts and in the *International Rheumatology News* not to mention the front pages of newspapers around the world. The Arthritis Foundation recognized the current antimycoplasma treatment in a special article by their "Unproven Remedies Committee," September 1981, and also in a Public Information Memo, June 1981, that told the public "there is no valid evidence that tetracycline can benefit rheumatoid arthritis victims."

Because the conclusions and recommendations in the NIH report are in direct conflict with information currently available from clinics and laboratories across the country and around the world (2, 11), it is considered vital for the millions of rheumatoid arthritis patients who have failed to benefit from the standard available therapy that this missing information be brought to the atten-

126

tion of the Congressional committees for necessary action.

Even though personal communications and letters to the editor were cited in the NIH report, for some unknown reason the report did not include references to recent published reports in the NIH library that emphasize the great need, the relevance, and the importance of antimycoplasmal research (7, 11, 13, 14, 16, 37).

For example:

Two prominent mycoplasma experts, supported by grants from NIH and the Arthritis Foundation (Cassell and Cole, 1981), reviewed the recent literature and reported in The New England Journal of Medicine the following conclusions:

1. "New information concerning the pathophysiology of mycoplasmas suggest that these organisms should be reevaluated as possible causes of arthritis in human beings."

2. In spite of inconsistent findings, "Compelling reasons still exist to suggest that the early speculations may be correct and that the role of mycoplasmas in rheumatoid arthritis deserves further investigation."

3. Thus not only is the mycoplasma hypothesis regarding rheumatoid arthritis possible, it even appears to be more plausible."

4. In view of the recent isolations of mycoplasmas directly from the joints of patients with arthritis, "It seems worthwhile to apply this information in a new search for mycoplasmas in chronic diseases."

Being microbiologists, these investigators have found animal models useful, but unfortunately not being clinicians, they have not applied their animal findings to the treatment of human rheumatoid arthritis as indicated.

Three prominent rheumatologists from the University of Colorado, Baylor College of Medicine, and the Mayo Clinic (Sharp, Lidsky and Duffy, 1982) (supported by grants from NIH, the Arthritis Foundation, Veterans Administration, and the Department of Health and Human Services) recently reported on the poor clinical responses in rheumatoid arthritis during gold therapy and raised some pertinent questions. "Why do less than half of the patients treated with gold therapy achieve remission?" (Or, why do more that half fail to benefit?) These investigators then raised the questions, "Are the effects of gold on experimental mycoplasma arthritis (in animals) relevant to its effectiveness in RA? Is rheumatoid arthritis an infection due to multiple strains of mycoplasmas that vary in gold sensitivity?" Apparently these authors know that gold is an antimycoplasma drug and that rheumatoid arthritis is the possible result of mycoplasma infection requiring a more effective and safer antimycoplasma drug than gold.

During a workshop on "Mycoplasmatales as agents of disease" at NIH (1971), the distinguished scientist and author Dr. Lewis Thomas (14) reviewed the use of gold salts in treating mycoplasmal diseases and stated that, "all this is obviously theoretical. I can imagine no practical application for gold in the management of any mycoplasmal disease since tetracycline and other antibiotics would be more effective and certainly far less hazardous."

"Because conventional antirheumatic medications may be associated with more toxicity than therapeutic benefits the search must continue for better and less harmful agents" (Arthritis Foundation 23rd Rheumatism Review, 1978). A review of the current disease-modifying drugs under investigation by the NIH (1983) indicates that the more dangerous agents (methotrexate and corticosteroids) are being pursued.

The NIH report also failed to mention that gold salts, the drug of first choice, has a high attrition or drop-out rate of about 30%/year and consequently very few chronic rheumatoid arthritis patients would benefit more than a few years. After a few years they would be started on the next more toxic drug (antimalarials or penicillamine), until finally the drug's side effects are worse than the disease (16-23).

Two prominent rheumatologists from Boston and Stanford have reported that "We cannot escape the conclusion that over the years several hundred million dollars has been expended on unproven monitoring procedures for gold toxicity, and that this sum cannot be shown to have purchased safety or health for even a single individual." (Liang and Fries, 1978).

The standard available drugs are especially dangerous for those 250,000 juveniles with rheumatoid arthritis who must face a lifetime of toxic drugs with a very high 5 to 20% mortality (24). By shutting the door to clinical trials of much safer antimycoplasma

128

drugs (antibiotics) that could indefinitely sustain control of their disease, many juveniles are being handed a lifetime sentence of pain and crippling without a fair trial.

The Arthritis Foundation claimed on public television and in their publications that "antibiotics do not help rheumatoid arthritis" (26). Congress and the Department of Health and Human Services should require the Arthritis Foundation to provide acceptable evidence to justify their claims that withhold a more effective and safer treatment. Their negative statement has ignored at least two favorable reports. 1. The utilization of the joint scan (scintigraphic) to provide objective favorable evidence of effectiveness of tetracycline that was presented at the International Congress of Rheumatology in 1977 and selected for special review in INFLO publication (27). 2. The more recent long term report was presented at the International Congress of Rheumatology in 1981 and at a university medical conference and published as a chapter in a medical textbook. This report provides significant information on the effectiveness of the antimycoplasma approach to treatment using five-year followup studies in a series of over 35 severe rheumatoid arthritis patients who were failures on the standard remedies (7).

Brown et al. (1966) were the first to report the localization of mycoplasma antibodies in the joint fluid of rheumatoid arthritis patients. This was later confirmed by Decker et al. (1975) in the swine model of mycoplasma-induced arthritis. Brown etal. (1969) were the first to report the successful control of spontaneous rheumatoid arthritis in a gorilla with parenteral (IV) tetracycline. This was later confirmed by veterinarians in several zoos and also by the successful control of mycoplasma-induced arthritis in the mouse model using parenteral tetracycline by Hannan (1977) and Taylor et al. (1978). Brown et al, (1949) were the first to report on the successful use of tetracycline in the treatment of humans with rheumatoid arthritis. This was later confirmed by Sanchez (1968) and more recently by several other doctors (personal communications).

These omissions of relevant information and other errors in content provide documented evidence that the request by Congress in Bill HR 7205 has not been fulfilled and that the report submitted by NIH to the Congress should be considered unacceptable.

Summary Statements:

1. Mycoplasmas are one of the most common known causes of arthritis in animals. In experimentally infected animals mycoplasmas cannot be readily isolated or detected after arthritis has progressed. Thus the required isolation of mycoplasmas from humans with long standing rheumatoid arthritis should be the exception to and not the rule as claimed in the NIH report.

2. It is also well known that tetracyclines and other antibiotics in low or oral doses (such as used in the negative 1971 study) do not readily inhibit the mycoplasmas infecting tissue cell cultures or experimental animals and humans except at the early stages. Even the mycoplasma vaccines have had limited success in animals and humans, often making humans worse. Apparently the mechanisms that limit mycoplasmas from ready isolation also prevent inhibition with antibiotics and vaccines and thus result in their lifetime persistence.

3. Because of mycoplasmas' ubiquitous or common occurrence in humans (and animals), neither their isolation nor detection of antibodies can be considered diagnostic or confirmatory evidence as they can be found in both symptomatic and asymptomatic hosts. However, if the rise and fall in mycoplasma antibody titers occurs in conjunction with a change in clinical symptoms or with treatment (as it often does), such serological evidence would certainly provide supportive prognostic information.

4. The experimentally induced mycoplasma arthritis in animals has been found to respond more favorably to parenteral (injected) antibiotics than routine oral therapy. Investigators in England and Canada concluded from their animal studies (5) that clinical trials with parenteral antibiotics should be tested in rheumatoid patients. Several gorillas (the closest animal to man) with spontaneous rheumatoid arthritis have responded favorably to antimycoplasma therapy after standard medications had failed (6).

5. The available information strongly supports the role of mycoplasma in rheumatoid disease (Clark et al. 1980), and several NIH-supported investigators have also concluded from their studies that mycoplasmas are the possible cause and should be studied. Three prominent rheumatologists (Sharp et al. 1982) suggested that the failure of gold therapy may be due to variations in myco-

130

plasma sensitivities, thus opening the door to more effective and safer antimycoplasma therapy.

When all of the currently available information is considered, both NIH and Congress will recognize the urgent need to initiate a long term clinical trial of antimycoplasma treatment as soon as possible. [Note: Congress (1989) appropriated the funds and NIH has initiated a clinical trial of tetracycline in RA patients.]

REFERENCES: (Used in the report to Congress)

1. Decker, JL and JA Barden. Immunological aspects of rheumatoid arthritis, in Rheumatology 6. Karger, Basel, 338-345, 1975.

2. Jansson Eli, et al. Cultivation of fastidious mycoplasmas from human arthritis. Z. Rheumatol. Zeitschrift fur Rheumatologie 42: 66-70, 1983.

3. Clark, HW and TMcP Brown. Another look at mycoplasmas. Arthritis Rheum. 19: 649-650, 1976.

4. Hannan, PCT. Sodium aurothiomalate, gold kerotinate and various tetracyclines in mycoplasma-induced arthritis in rodents. J. Med. Microbiol. 10: 87-102, 1977.

5. Taylor GD, Taylor-Robinson D, and EC Keystone. Effect of lymecycline on *Mycoplasma pulmonis*-induced arthritis in mice. Br. J. Exp. Pathol. 59: 204-121, 1978.

6. Brown TMcP, HW Clark and JS Bailey. Rheumatoid arthritis in the gorilla: A study of mycoplasma-host interaction in pathogenesis and treatment, in Comparative Pathology of Zoo Animals, eds. and R J Montali and G Migaki. Smithsonian Institution Press, 259-266, 1980.

7. Brown TMcP, HW Clark and JS Bailey. Antimycoplasma approach to the mechanism and the control of rheumatoid disease, in Inflammatory Diseases and Copper, ed. JRJ Sorenson. The Humana Press, 391-407, 1982.

131

8.   Harwick HJ, GM Kalmanson and B Gazel. Effect of antibiotics on Mycoplasma pulmonis arthritis in mice. Abstract from 14th Interscience Conference on Antimicrobial Agents and Chemotherapy, 47, 1974.

9.   Nocard E, E Roux, et al. Le microbe de la peripneumonie. Ann. Inst. Pasteur, Paris, 12: 240-262, 1898.

10.   Robinson LB, TMcP Brown and RH Wichelhausen. Studies on the effect of erythromycin and antimalarial compounds on pleuropneumonia-like organisms. Antibiot. and Chemother. 9: 111-114, 1959.

11.   Cassell, G and BC Cole. Mycoplasmas as agents of human disease. N. Engl. J. Med. 304: 80-89, 1981.

12.   Hayflick L. The role of mycoplasmas in human arthritis. The Kroc Foundation Medical Research Programs, 45, 1981.

13.   Sharp JT , MD Lidsky and J Duffy. Clinical responses during gold therapy for rheumatoid arthritis. Arthritis Rheum. 25: 540-549, 1982.

14.   Thomas L. Workshop on the mycoplasmatales as agents of disease, summary discussion. J. Infect. Dis. 127 Supplement: 87-88, 1973.

15.   Arthritis Foundation: 23rd Rheumatism Review. Arthritis Rheum. 28, 1978.

16.   Bunch TW and JD O'Duffy. Disease-modifying drugs for progressive rheumatoid arthritis. Mayo Clinic Proc. 55: 161-179, 1980.

17.   Stein HB, AC Patterson, et al. Adverse effects of D-penicillamine in rheumatoid arthritis. Ann. of Intern. Med. 92: 24-29, 1980.

18.   Weiss AS, JA Markenson, et al. Toxicity of D-penicillamine in

rheumatoid arthritis. Am. J. Med. 64: 114-120, 1978.

19.   Anastassiades TP.   Remission-inducing drugs in rheumatoid arthritis.   Canada Med. Assoc. J. 122: 405-415, 1980.

20.   Sharp JT , Lidsky MD and J Duffy, et al.   Comparison of two dosage schedules of gold salts in the treatment of rheumatoid arthritis.   Arthritis Rheum. 20: 1179-1187, 1977.

21.   Stafford BT and WH Crosby.   Late onset of gold-induced thrombocytopenia.   JAMA 239: 50-51, 1978.

22.   Gibbons RB.   Complications of chrysotherapy–a review of recent studies.   Arch. Intern. Med. 139: 343-356, 1979.

23.   Davis P.   Undesirable effects of gold salts.   J Rheumatol. Suppl. 5: 18-23, 1979.

24.   Stoeber E.   Corticosteroid treatment of juvenile chronic polyarthritis over 22 years.   Eur. J. Pediatr. 121: 141-147, 1976.

25.   Mitchell DM and JF Fries.   An analysis of the American Rheumatism Association criteria for rheumatoid arthritis.   Arthritis Rheum. 25: 481-487, 1982.

26.   Arthritis Foundation.   Basic Facts, p. 6, 1978.

27.   Brown TMcP and HW Clark.   Rheumatoid inflammation. INFLO, Vol. 11, 1-2. The Upjohn Company, 1978.

28.   Thomas L.   New directions in arthritis research.   Arthritis Foundation Report, 1973.

29.   Gumpel JM.   Deaths associated with gold treatment: A reassessment.   Brit. Med. J. 2: 215-216, 1978.

30.   Ward JR.   New approaches to trials of antirheumatic drugs in rheumatoid arthritis.   J Clin. Pharmacol. 15: 367-372, 1975.

31. Fries JF and MC Britton. Some problems in the interpretation of clinical trials. J. of Rheumatol. S2: 61-66, 1976.

32. Forestier J. L'aurotherapie dans les rheumatismes chroniques. Bull. Mem. Soc. Med. Hosp., Paris 53: 323-327, 1929.

33. Sabin AB and J Warren. The curative effect of certain gold compounds on experimental proliferative, chronic arthritis in mice. J. Bacteriol. 40: 832, 1940.

34. Liang MH and JF Fries. Containing costs in chronic disease: Monitoring strategies in gold therapy on rheumatoid arthritis. Editorial, J. Rheumatol. 5: 241-243, 1978.

35. Brown TMcP et al. Comparative aspects of rheumatoid arthritis in the gorilla and man. XVth International Congress of Rheumatology, 1981 (abstract).

36. Arthritis Foundation. Mycoplasma/tetracycline therapy. Public Information Memo, June 26, 1981.

37. Cole BC and JR Ward. Mycoplasmas as arthritogenic agents, in The Mycoplasmas, Vol. II, eds. Tully JG and Wittcomb RF, Academic Press, 367-395, 1979.

38. Brown TMcP, RH Wichelhausen, LB Robinson and WR Merchant. The In vivo action of aureomycin on pleuropneumonia-like organisms associated with various rheumatoid diseases. J. Lab. Clin. Med. 34: 1404-1410, 1949.

39. Skinner M, ES Cathcort, JA Mills and RS Pinals. Tetracycline in the treatment of rheumatoid arthritis. Arthritis Rheum. 14: 727-735, 1971.

40. Sanchez I. Tetracycline treatment in rheumatoid arthritis and other rheumatic diseases. Brazil Med. 82: 22-31, 1968.

41. Clark HW, JS Bailey and TMcP Brown. Properties support-

ing the role of mycoplasmas in rheumatoid arthritis. Reviews of Infectious Diseases, Vol. 4: S238, 1982.

Published In: HEARINGS, Part 9, 714-741, 1983
before the U.S. House of Representatives
Appropriations Subcommittee for the Dept. HHS.

* * *

The following Chapter VIII report (less attachments), together with the author's bracketed comments, provides further evidence both for and against the support of anti-mycoplasma therapy and thus provides the public with current expert knowledge of arthritis.

Chapter VIII

National Institutes of Health
Report on Mycoplasma, Antimycoplasma
Therapy, and Rheumatoid Arthritis

Introduction
In its report on the Fiscal Year 1983 budget for the Department of Health and Human Services, the Senate Committee on Appropriations stated:

> "The Committee wishes to be kept apprised of the Institute's research into mycoplasma-related causes of rheumatoid arthritis. The Committee expects the Institute to examine relevant clinical data and report back within the year its assessment of whatever lines of inquiry may be suggested. Such a review should take into account the possible importance of duration of treatment as a variable in evaluating the mycoplasma perspective."

(Senate Report No. 97-680, page 41)
The following report has been prepared by the National Institute of Arthritis, Diabetes, and Digestive and Kidney Diseases (NIAD-DK) of the National Institutes of Health (NIH), Department of Health and Human Services (HHS), in response to this request.

Methods
This report combines and summarizes the findings of two recent technical reports on research in mycoplasmas and arthritis. The First Technical Report (attachment A) was based on a previous literature review

prepared by the National Institute of Arthritis, Diabetes, and Digestive and Kidney Diseases (NIADDK) and submitted to the House Appropriations Committee in February 1983 [see above report]. Modifications of the February 1983 report have been made in attachment A (1) to incorporate the latest scientific evidence; (2) to take into account comments submitted by the Arthritis Institute of the National Hospital, Arlington, Virginia [see above report]; and (3) to respond specifically to the Senate's concern about clinical data on mycoplasma and duration of treatment as a variable in evaluating the mycoplasma perspective. The NIADDK literature review was prepared with the advice of experts in several fields. Scientific papers covered were primarily those that had been published in peer reviewed journals, that is, journals that require review and comment by fellow researchers prior to publication.

The Second Technical Report (attachment B) was prepared by an expert panel of rheumatologists convened by the National Arthritis Advisory Board (NAAB) [*] at the request of NIADDK. The Board, which is comprised of eminent, national scientific and lay leaders, is mandated by law to review and evaluate national efforts in research, treatment, education and training to combat the many forms of arthritis. At its September 1983 meeting the full Board discussed and approved the report prepared by the expert panel. *Appointed by the Secretary of HHS.

[According to the National Arthritis Act of 1975, as the National Advisors, the success or failure of finding the cause and the cure of rheumatoid disorders rests in their hands. In their report to NIH, they failed to provide a more promising direction while devaluing the "untested" antimycoplasma approach.]

Rheumatoid Arthritis—Research, Therapy

Rheumatoid arthritis (RA) is one of the most prevalent and potentially crippling forms of arthritis. It causes heat, swelling and pain in the joints, as well as weakness, fatigue and general malaise. There is wide variation in its course and degree of severity; patients range from those with mild and sometimes temporary disease to those with significant pain and deformity. The disease tends to be chronic, disabling and irregular—it can flare up suddenly and thereafter go into remission.

138

Causes

Although there is no fully established theory as to why rheumatoid arthritis occurs, research into its causes and development is entering a new phase of increased productivity. Several areas of study are involved (these are reviewed in much greater detail in the NAAB report).

(1) Genetic factors are clearly implicated. Such factors may be related to how a person's immune system functions and may explain why some people are affected and some are not.
[Genetic factors are not a cause but predisposing susceptibility conditions giving rise to multiple varieties and severity of arthritis.]

(2) Many investigators are studying the role of triggering agents that may set off the immuno-inflammatory process. They believe a variety of such agents may be involved, including substances within the body, as well as external agents, such as different viruses, bacteria, or mycoplasmas.
[The agents should be persistent (lifelong), latent, and infectious, yet noncontagious, and not a one-shot trigger.]

(3) Greater understanding has been gained of the immune system and its response to "foreign" substances, particularly the complex process of inflammation.
[The immune response and the resulting inflammation are the results of the unknown foreign infectious agent and thus not the cause.]

(4) In rheumatoid arthritis, chronic inflammation can lead to the destruction of joint cartilage and underlying bone.
[Yes, but symptoms are the results of the disease and not the cause.]

As the NAAB report points out, research indicates that rheumatoid arthritis is a complex and heterogeneous disease. Indeed, it may be that several different combinations of factors described above could all result in the set of symptoms and signs that comprise RA.
[Many factors, especially the infinite genetic differences, contribute to the resulting variable symptoms, but what are the causes?]

Treatment

Current therapy for rheumatoid arthritis is not ideal. As the NAAB report states, "We have no predictably efficacious therapy for rheumatoid arthritis at the present time." The report explains, however, that research has expanded the arsenal of therapies for rheumatoid arthritis considerably in recent years; a host of non-steroidal anti-inflammatory drugs is available and, for more severe cases, the stronger "disease modifying" drugs.

[Most of which are now being reported as not modifying the course of rheumatoid arthritis.]

The NAAB report also lists the experimental therapies currently being evaluated by researchers; these include cytotoxic drugs, total lymphocyte irradiation, leukopheresis and plasmapheresis. *[These procedures are very limited and extremely costly, have far greater risks, and have not been shown to modify the disease course.]*

The NAAB report stresses that, as new therapies develop, "current practice and discipline suggest that double-blind controlled studies are the only appropriate method of confirming efficacy of test drugs in rheumatoid arthritis. In such trials, two groups of patients are compared. One group receives the test drug, and the other receives a placebo (an inactive preparation) or standard drug (e.g., aspirin, in the case of rheumatoid arthritis trials). To avoid bias, none of the patients or the health professionals who treat them know which patients receive the experimental therapy. A control group is particularly important, says the NAAB expert panel: "The placebo effect of skilled, confident and co-passionate deliverers of health care can never be underestimated (A placebo effect is the response of patients to what they perceive is a genuine therapy)." *[The invasive experimental therapies cited above have never been double-blind tested. A placebo effect would hardly apply to experimental animals, such as a gorilla, nor last more than a few months and thus the need for long term-trials, which would soon become intolerable and unethical.]*

Mycoplasmas

Both the NAAB report and the NIADDK review explain that mycoplasmas are tiny organisms similar to bacteria in some respects,

140

but different from them in others. Some characteristics of mycoplasmas are listed below and described in greater detail in the two appended reports, particularly part III of the NAAB report. Many of these characteristics can make it challenging to study mycoplasmas and determine their role in disease.

Another look at mycoplasmas would find that they are markedly different from bacteria and viruses.]

(1)   Mycoplasmas lack a cell wall and are therefore nonsusceptible to the penicillins. Mycoplasmas are susceptible to antibiotics such as tetracyclines and erythromycin.

[Also gold salts, Plaquenil, and copper-penicillamine, and unlike bacteria and viruses firmly attach to joint and other specific tissues.]

(2)   They are ubiquitous. Some 65 species are known. They occur in nature, can grow in cell cultures in laboratories (and, in fact, often contaminate cell cultures), and can grow within man, animals, birds, arthropods, and plants. Mycoplasmas can cause certain diseases in animals and humans. They are also normally present in both (as are many bacteria) without causing disease.

[The widespread contamination of cell cultures was first reported by our lab. Mycoplasma-infected humans, animals, trees, and plants are all effectively treated with tetracycline.]

(3)   They are small enough to be mistaken for viruses.

[Except that they do not require living cells for growth and are inhibited by antibiotics.]

(4)   Seen under a microscope, they easily can be confused with cellular debris. They also attach to the surface of cells in tissue culture and samples of pathological tissue, which may explain why they are hard to get rid of in cell cultures and infected animals.

[Without a cell wall mycoplasmas are highly pleomorphic. Also in humans, mycoplasmas are difficult to isolate and are poorly responsive to antibiotics and vaccines.]

(5)   They are "fastidious" in that they require specialized media to grow in a laboratory. At the same time, some of the ingre-

dients of these media are sometimes contaminated with outside sources of mycoplasmas.
[As are many specimens, tissue cell cultures, and laboratory animals that require special expert handling techniques.]

(6)   Rather stringent criteria have been defined for researchers to identify mycoplasma species.   Unless these are followed, investigators cannot strictly say they have found a particular species or that what they have found are really mycoplasmas.
[In order to isolate and identify mycoplasmas, they must first be adapted to the artificial culture conditions, which can alter some of their natural properties.]

Mycoplasmas and Disease
Both appended reports explain that in humans, mycoplasmas cause respiratory infections and have been associated with genitourinary infections.   In fact, as the NIADDK review points out, they were once called pleuropneumonia-like organisms (PPLO) because one mycoplasma species causes atypical pneumonia.
[Mycoplasmas have also been reported and classified under Mycoplasma Arthritis. The first strain was isolated from cattle with pleuropneumonia and arthritis in 1898. Subsequent isolates were referred to as PPLO. A viral-like strain isolated from patients with atypical pneumonia was recently identified and named Mycoplasma pneumoniae.]

Studies have shown that mycoplasmas also cause joint inflammation (arthritis) in mice, rats, swine, cattle, sheep, goats and domestic fowl.   According to the NAAB report, however, there is no convincing evidence that mycoplasmas cause arthritis in gorillas, particularly not rheumatoid arthritis, which is a disease restricted to humans.
[Why? see below.]

Both reports make the point, however, that some forms of animal mycoplasma arthritis are similar to rheumatoid arthritis and are used as research models for human arthritis.
[Is or isn't rheumatoid arthritis found in animals? Only the gorillas (great apes) were found to be infected with the human mycoplasma

142

strains and are immunologically related to humans making them the closest animal model of human rheumatoid arthritis.]

The NAAB report points out that strong evidence supporting the role of mycoplasmas in animal arthritis exists. Investigators have been able to isolate the suspected mycoplasmas from arthritic animals, grow them in culture and then reproduce the illness by inoculating subcultures of the organism into normal animals. Though ethics do not permit such inoculation of humans, many investigators have attempted the first step—trying to isolate and culture mycoplasmas from arthritis patients-as will be described further.

[NIH has inoculated mycoplasma into human test subjects. The mycoplasma initiates an infectious response of atypical pneumonia, which apparently can progress to various immunologic disorders such as arthritis and paralysis as well as pneumonia.]

Mycoplasmas and Arthritis in Man

Since the 1930's, there has been significant scientific interest in mycoplasmas as a cause of arthritis in man. As both the NAAB report and the NIADDK review describe at length, a considerable number of researchers the world over have looked for a variety of mycoplasma species in samples from the joints of patients with rheumatoid arthritis, Reiter's syndrome, venereal arthritis, psoriatic arthritis, and other diseases. From all these studies, there have been numerous positive reports (i.e., of studies in which mycoplasmas were found) as well as negative reports (of studies in which mycoplasmas were not found). The NAAB expert panel points out that "no unequivocal, confirmed isolations have been made from the synovial fluid or tissue of patients with rheumatoid arthritis".

[As one of the expert panel members previously reported, the mycoplasma or infectious agent could be localized at some distant site and not localized in the inflamed synovial tissue tested. It is also well known that mycoplasmas are not readily isolated from the experimentally inoculated arthritic animal model even though antibodies persist. Although mycoplasmas can be detected in tissue cell cultures, they resist isolation.]

The NAAB panel further explains: "A large number of reported isolations are considered doubtful or of unknown validity, primarily because the organisms have not been subcultured or have not been appropriately identified, because the investigators have utilized cell cultures or other reagents that are frequently contaminated, or because they have depended entirely on morphologic identification (i.e., identification by the use of a microscope) under circumstances that are regularly associated with large numbers of artifacts."

[Many positive isolations have been made under valid controlled conditions, which should not be compared with erroneous results of inexperienced investigators.]

To quote the NAAB report further, "if studies in which technical factors surrounding reported isolations are completely discounted then there is no evidence for a mycoplasma etiology of rheumatoid arthritis. If one considers that some or all of the reported isolations may be correct, then several possibilities emerge." These possibilities given by the NAAB panel are:

(1) Mycoplasmas may occasionally infect patients who already have rheumatoid arthritis producing an infectious (mycoplasma) arthritis.

(2) RA may be more than one disease process and mycoplasmas may be one of many causes.
[What are the other causes, bacteria and viruses? Perhaps rheumatoid arthritis is one disease mechanism with many targets and individual variations.]

(3) Although mycoplasmas may initiate RA, their persistence is not necessary to maintaining disease activity and progression.
[If not, what turns off and on the disease at infrequent and irregular intervals? Mycoplasmas can remain dormant in tissues as a neutralized living irritant and foreign antigen.]

Both the NAAB report and the NIADDK review also note

144

that many investigators have done immunological studies to look for antibodies to mycoplasmas in the blood of patients. Such studies are designed largely to show if the organisms are or were at one time present. According to the NAAB expert panel, results to date from these immunological studies do not suggest a role for known mycoplasma species in rheumatoid arthritis.

[Investigators in Finland found a very high incidence of mycoplasma antibodies in their rheumatoid arthritis patients. A four-fold rise in mycoplasma antibody titer has been associated with a flare or worsening in RA patients. The expert panel and NIH should know that some RA patients do not produce antibodies or that in the presence of the anti-antibody rheumatoid factor, a negative mycoplasma antibody test does not rule them out.]

Current and Future Research on Mycoplasmas

The NAAB report's consideration of mycoplasma research found it to be a flourishing scientific area. Moreover, both traditional and new investigative methods hold promise for enhancing identification of these organisms. Improved microbiological techniques, including new culture methods, are under investigation by several talented research groups. In addition, new techniques that have revolutionized molecular biology over the past six years or so—monoclonal antibodies (to locate mycoplasma antigens), cloning (of specific mycoplasma genes), and DNA probes (to look for evidence of mycoplasmas)—may be maturing in ways that foster clinical and diagnostic applications in patients with rheumatoid arthritis.

[As yet, most of these new techniques have not been thoroughly tested or applied to experimental animals or rheumatoid arthritis patients. Why continue to withhold safe and effective tetracycline therapy while waiting for someone to prove the infectious cause of rheumatoid arthritis?]

Clinical Data on Antimycoplasma therapy for Rheumatoid Arthritis

The Senate has specifically requested that NIH examine relevant clinical data regarding the mycoplasma perspective. To quote the NAAB expert panel, "Does long-term antibiotic therapy affect the course of rheumatoid arthritis? This is a valid question to pose, because we have no predictably efficacious therapy for rheumatoid

145

arthritis at the present time. There are several pieces (perhaps unrelated) of information that frame the logic behind the question."

(1) There are a number of animal models of arthritis in which the process is caused by mycoplasmas or some other microbial agent.
[Arthritic animals have been successfully treated with antibiotics, especially intravenous tetracycline.]

(2) There have been many reports over the past three decades of mycoplasmas having been isolated on rare occasions from patients with rheumatoid arthritis.
[Sometimes not so rare. Investigators in Finland reported 100%.]

(3) Certain drugs (notably gold salts), which are generally considered useful in the therapy of rheumatoid arthritis, are known to inhibit mycoplasma growth.
[Also hydroxychloroquine and bee venom.]

(4) Antibiotics, such as tetracyclines and erythromycin, are known to be quite effective in treatment of human mycoplasma infection (such as Mycoplasma pneumoniae).
[Wrong, only partially effective unless given early and preferably intravenously, as mycoplasmas continue to be shed.]

(5) Anecdotal reports by Dr. Thomas McPherson Brown and colleagues at the Arthritis Institute, National Hospital, Arlington, Virginia, suggest that long-term (one-to-five-year) antibiotic therapy may be beneficial in rheumatoid arthritis patients.
[Although the Arthritis Foundation has reported that "antibiotics were of no benefit in RA," many doctors around the world have found tetracyclines to be very beneficial and safe for their rheumatoid arthritis patients.]

The NAAB report continues, "In spite of these clues and of the intense interest of microbiologists, rheumatologists and the public we must ask a second question, what are the scientific data?"

146

[How scientific are the current empirical and palliative RA ther-
apies (gold salts, penicillamine, methotrexate, etc) should be the
first question.]

Both the NAAB report and the NIADDK review identified only one controlled clinical trial of antimycoplasma therapy for rheumatoid arthritis, a study reported in 1971 and referenced by both reports. To quote the NAAB expert panel: "After an exhaustive review of the world literature there can be found only one objectively reported study in a peer reviewed journal dealing with antibiotic therapy in rheumatoid arthritis (Skinner et al., 1971). That study on a small number of patients treated for one year with daily doses of tetracycline (250 mg.) failed to show any therapeutic efficacy above the control group. There are no other scientifically credible studies on this topic at the clinical level."
[As discussed above, this very small study of 13 patients was a classical
Type II statistical error and can hardly be termed scientifically credi-
ble data, any more than Dr. Brown's retrospective study of 98 patients
treated over a 5-year period (ILAR 1985. See Brown et al. 1949 and
1951).]

Both reports also addressed the reports of Dr. Brown and coworkers mentioned in (5) above. Dr. Brown's reports describe favorable responses of patients to antimycoplasma therapy. The NAAB report notes, however, that his reports "are of only anecdotal interest," that is they provide descriptions, but offer no scientific evidence. The information Dr. Brown's reports provide is of a clinical nature, but is not comparable to a clinical trial. That is, there is no control (comparison) group, and, "in the patients treated" says the NAAB report, "none of the results of criteria recommended for inclusion in a controlled double-blind study have been published. The powerful placebo effect of attention, optimism and enthusiasm of good physicians has been ignored."
[The experts should know that attention, optimism, and enthusiasm
are essential ingredients of good medicine and the favorable responses,
even anecdotal, are of vital interest to the many arthritic patients who
have failed to benefit on other treatment.]

In particular, the 1982 article by Dr. Brown and coworkers, which is referenced and addressed by both appended technical reports does not, as the NIADDK review describes, (a) "provide detailed clinical information about these patients with which to substantiate the diagnosis of RA"; (b) define the "standard treatment" to which these patients are reported to be refractory; or (c) define the "mean clinical Index", although "there are well-defined and broadly tested indexes and methods of assessing the clinical activity of RA as well as laboratory tests which can be used for this purpose."

[Rather than examine Brown's patients' charts, the panel of experts chose to refute his 40 plus years of rheumatology experience, his ability to diagnose rheumatoid arthritis, his knowledge of standard drugs, and his ability to measure clinical changes. Brown is not the first medical pioneer to be criticized by his peers.]

The NIADDK review goes on to say that, "without appropriate control patients (i.e., those who do not receive tetracycline), it is difficult to conclude that the perceived benefit is due to the antimycoplasma therapy."

[Since most of the patients had failed on gold, plaquenil, and other so-called disease-modifying drugs, they are thus bonafide cross-over controls, comparing years on one drug with years on another.]

Duration of Treatment

The Senate has also specifically requested that in preparing this report, NIH consider the possible importance of duration of treatment as a variable in addressing the mycoplasma perspective. This aspect is addressed by both appended reports. The NIADDK review states that, "other than Dr. Brown's and coworkers' report of their experiences using the antimycoplasma approach to treating humans with rheumatoid arthritis and gorillas with arthritis resembling rheumatoid arthritis, no support in the medical literature could be found for the rationale of extending tetracycline therapy for rheumatoid arthritis patients to five years."

[There are many valid reasons—the most appropriate being that 90 to 95% of the rheumatoid arthritis patients fail to benefit and stay on gold and other available therapies for five years (Fig. 1 & 2 p 158-59).

148

Successful long term (48 months) controlled tetracycline trials for other skeletal disorders have been reported by other investigators.]

The NAAB report points to a "flaw" in the arguments of Dr. Brown and colleagues: "It is that anti-infectious therapy which attains cidal ("killing") tissue concentrations for an agent that causes and sustains a disease such as rheumatoid arthritis should have beneficial effects notable within a year, particularly because appropriate antibiotic levels can be reached in tissues within days."

[The NAAB report is the one seriously flawed, as tetracycline is not a mycoplasma "killing" agent but rather inhibits protein synthesis and growth by nucleic acid binding. The appropriate (inhibiting) antibiotic levels for mycoplasmas in a cell free media (test tube) do not eradicate them in tissue cell cultures. Unless treated early, even experimental mycoplasma animal models do not respond to tetracycline and require intravenous therapy (see above description of tetracyclines' multiple actions). Tetracyclines are more than antibiotics and can act as anti-inflammatories as well as immunosuppressives, antioxidants, and antimetalloenzymes such as collagenase. In some patients, beneficial results may occur in less than one year but are not sustained. The bactericidal antibiotic level of tetracycline in tissues and blood is only one measure of its activity.]

Recommendations
The recommendations of the NAAB report and the NIADDK review concerned further investigations of mycoplasmas and arthritis and possibly of antimycoplasma therapy.

Recommendations Against a Large Clinical Trial
Both the NAAB and the NIADDK review affirm the possibility that mycoplasmas may have a role in the development of rheumatoid arthritis. The NAAB panel states that "We must take seriously the possibility that they (mycoplasmas) cause arthritis in humans." Neither report, however, recommends a large, clinical trial of antimycoplasma therapy.

The NAAB report states, "This Panel . . . can find no compelling evidence at this time to initiate a large, costly clinical trial of antibiotic therapy in RA." The NAAB panel also states, "Reports

149

of antimycoplasma agents being efficacious in treatment of RA . . .
are not sufficient to warrant a broad-scale study of these drugs in
RA." Says the NIADDK review, "The weight of current evidence .
. . does not warrant the initiation of a large-scale, long-term, multicenter clinical trial of tetracycline treatment of rheumatoid arthritis at this time."

*[Even though the experts say they should take the mycoplasma cause
seriously, they completely refused to acknowledge and recommend taking the initial first step, i.e., a pilot clinical trial of tetracycline therapy. They hold the purse strings. Who or what are they waiting for? Ten
years later (1994), NIH made sufficient funds available to investigate tetracycline therapy and the mycoplasma cause of rheumatoid
arthritis.]*

Recommendations for Further Clinical Studies on Mycoplas-mas and Arthritis and Possible Antimycoplasma therapy

Both reports make additional suggestions for future research in mycoplasmas and arthritis. The NIADDK review points out that research using mycoplasma induced arthritis in animals as a model for
human arthritis is useful and is continuing. Indeed, NIH, through
the NIADDK, is supporting and conducting arthritis research using these animal models.

*[If animal models are so useful, why haven't they benefitted human
arthritis? The tetracycline therapy used for arthritic animals has not
been supported or adequately tested in humans by NIH.]*

The NAAB report on mycoplasmas and arthritis concludes
by suggesting that the leadership of NIH consider two sequential clinical studies. First, "If NIH program directors consider it appropriate,
a multicenter study of 100 patients with active rheumatoid arthritis
(less than two years duration and hopefully within six months of diagnosis) and 100 patients with nonrheumatoid chronic arthritis could
be developed. Synovial tissue could be obtained via multiple samples
using closed needle biopsy after institutional approval by Human Studies
Committees. Samples would be frozen and sent to at least two laboratories for mycoplasma studies." It should be noted, however, that
any ethical issues concerning the removal of tissue and blood samples
from these patients would have to be addressed in the design of this

study. The report further states, "The odds of recovery of mycoplasma organisms or detection of antigenic material derived from them would be increased greatly over finding organisms or their trace in synovial fluid. Synovial biopsy via needle is a benign procedure in the hands of practiced rheumatologists. It is likely that many samples can be obtained from biopsies obtained at arthroscopic examination for purposes of diagnosis."

[This recommended study is highly unethical, especially when the proposed techniques and procedures have not been previously tested on experimental animals with mycoplasma arthritis. As a member of our hospital's Institutional Review Board, I certainly could not approve of the proposed human study until demonstrated in animal models.]

The NAAB report goes on to suggest that, "A second study, to be considered after completion of the first and only if significant numbers of biopsies yield positive results, would be a double-blind treatment trial...inclusion in a treatment protocol should be reserved for those who had mycoplasmas demonstrated in joint fluid or synovium by standardized, modern techniques as described previously in the NAAB report. Patients who were culture or antigen-positive would be randomized (half in therapy and half in a control group), put on long-term antibiotic therapy (dose to be determined), and evaluated by multiple criteria. After a course of therapy, repeat tissue biopsies would be obtained for culture and antigen search.

[Finding a microbial agent in any patient's joint should automatically require antibiotic therapy, preferably intraarticularly and certainly not a placebo.]

The expert panel also stated that, "This method, a double-blind study only of culture or antigen positive patients proven to have mycoplasma infection in joints, will be the only way to link antimycoplasma therapy with efficacy in the complex and heterogeneous disease that is rheumatoid arthritis."

[The experts should realize that such a very costly and questionable study would provide no proof of mycoplasma etiology. The mycoplasma agent could be deposited in some other tissues of the complex and heterogeneous disease and certainly is not the best way to test the efficacy and safety of tetracycline therapy in rheumatoid arthritis.]

Conclusions

After considering the scientific evidence presented in the reports of the NAAB expert panel and the NIAADK literature review, the Institute concurs with the findings and recommendations submitted. The Institute agrees that further research on the role of mycoplasmas in rheumatoid arthritis is appropriate, and it is making plans to initiate the biopsy study recommended by NAAB for its consideration.

[NIH may state that research on the role of mycoplasmas in rheumatoid arthritis is appropriate but they did not fund our approved mycoplasma research grant applications. After their report was submitted, NIH invited viral, bacterial, and mycoplasma experts to a workshop to discuss the ways and means of identifying the infectious cause of early rheumatoid arthritis. At that time (1985), many of the new techniques proposed in their recommendations were not readily available.]

To quote the NAAB expert panel:

"It appears that rheumatoid arthritis is a disorder involving multiple causative factors. It also seems likely that if mycoplasmas can cause RA it is probable that in only a small percentage of RA patients would mycoplasmas be involved etiologically."

* * *

Fortunately, someone saw the serious flaws and highly questionable procedures in the recommended clinical trial of tetracycline in mycoplasma-infected rheumatoid arthritis patients and it was not pursued. However, the fallacious and prejudicial NIH report did result in their not approving and thus withholding support for our two proposed clinical trials of tetracycline efficacy in rheumatoid arthritis patients.

Chapter IX

Further Comments On Rheumatoid Arthritis Therapy

T he NAAB expert panel report and NIADDK literature review used by NIH completely circumvented the primary issue and question of whether long-term tetracycline therapy affects the course of rheumatoid arthritis. More specifically, they did not compare the long-term use of the much safer and less toxic antibiotics with the ineffective therapy currently being used and dropped (See Figs 1 and 2). Most of the drugs for treating rheumatoid arthritis are used empirically—that is, not directed toward eliminating any particular cause, such as infectious—and thus are primarily symptomatic and temporarily palliative. Why didn't the panel of experts also include antibiotics as another alternative empirical therapy? The successful tetracycline treatment of rheumatoid arthritis patients with and without positive mycoplasma tests would still not prove or disprove that mycoplasmas are the cause of rheumatoid arthritis.

It seems that NIH's main consideration should be to search for and test safer and more effective therapies based on any plausible evidence, no matter how limited. We could also ask what compelling evidence supported the costly clinical trials and approval of the copper complexing penicillamine in the 1970's which is now too toxic to use. Or we could ask what compelling evidence supported the more recent costly clinical trials of methotrexate, an ex-

153

tremely toxic liver damaging anti-cancer and immunosuppressive drug. So why do the experts not want to test the safer antibiotic tetracyclines in rheumatoid arthritis an inflammatory disease of suspected infectious origin? As a connective tissue and collagen vascular disorder, with elevated amounts of destructive collagenase activity, it would seem most likely that the inhibitory tetracycline therapy would certainly benefit the RA patients and perhaps even stop the disease.

Fortunately, reports by Decker (1984) and by Clark (1988, 1989) make the NAAB and NIH recommendations obsolete while reinforcing the mycoplasmas as a most probable cause of rheumatoid arthritis and consequently antimycoplasma therapy.

Evolving Concepts of Cause and Treatment.

In October 1983, rheumatologists at NIH held a combined staff conference to review and discuss "Rheumatoid Arthritis: Evolving Concepts of Pathogenesis and Treatment" (Decker, 1984). Holding this conference may have been coincidental to the Congressional Appropriation Committee's request for the NIH reports and should be viewed as coming from a different group of experts on the cause and treatment of rheumatoid arthritis. Two compelling reasons for the conference were the enormous size of the problem, with 1 percent of all humans having rheumatoid arthritis and the lingering fact that the cause of the disease is still unknown and its treatment is very unsatisfactory. The chronic inflammatory disease (unlike acute animal arthritis) is characterized by periods of remission (good days) and exacerbation (bad days) for unknown reasons. The NIH doctors believe that the disease represents the results of a genetically controlled host immune response to an undefined causative stimulus. The current hypotheses of causative factors that drive the persistent rheumatoid disease were listed as (1) deposition of immune complex in tissues, (2) persistence of mycoplasmas, (3) chronic viral infections, (4) deposition of bacterial debris, (5) anticollagen antibodies, and (6) abnormal stimulation of WBCs.

Although all of these agents are known to promote arthritis separately and perhaps collectively, the persistence of the viable neutralized mycoplasmas could explain both the chronicity of rheuma-

154

toid arthritis and the disease-modifying effects of the standard DMARs as well as the tetracycline antibiotics. As mentioned above, NIH held a national conference 27 years earlier in 1966 on "The Relationship of Mycoplasma to Rheumatoid Arthritis and Related Disease." Only two references to mycoplasma arthritis were cited in the recent conference while totally omitting any reference to the reports on antimycoplasma therapy. Citing mycoplasmas as a persistent factor in rheumatoid tissues at their NIH staff conference, which was published in the Annals of Internal Medicine, the staff failed to reference any of mycoplasma's 40 plus years of evolving concepts. Although frequently used by NIH, the experimental animal models such as swine arthritis do not have all the features of human rheumatoid arthritis. The NIH staff should have at least considered the evolving therapeutic probes that are aimed at eliminating the hypothetical or suspected causative factors and not just the resulting symptoms. Why not test tetracycline in humans knowing that it benefits the animal models and is less toxic and costly than gold therapy?

The NIH staff showed that the mechanism of inflammatory destruction of synovial connective tissue, characteristic of rheumatoid arthritis, was produced by the activated enzyme collagenase from the WBCs. All of this starts with the attachment of a foreign antigen (such as mycoplasmas or an immune complex) to the tissues. In discussing evolving concepts of treatment, the NIH staff did not indicate the potential use of antibiotics, even though persistent mycoplasmas and bacteria were considered possible factors. The fact that tetracyclines are also immunosuppressants and potent collagenase inhibitors that have been used to control inflammatory tissue disorders would seem to indicate their additional therapeutic roles.

Both the NAAB panel of experts and NIH previously reported that "Because we know that mycoplasmas can cause arthritis in many animals, and because we know that they do cause acute and chronic diseases in humans (in lungs and the genitourinary tract), we must take seriously the possibility that mycoplasmas can cause arthritis in humans." The question remains whether they also cause chronic rheumatoid disorders. The expert panel said they could find no compelling evidence at that time to initiate a large, costly

155

clinical trial of antibiotic therapy in rheumatoid arthritis. The panel concluded that "Current and evolving techniques give us hope that broad studies of synovial tissue may reveal a causative organism," which seems to be the same old needle-in-the-haystack approach. Using some of the newer techniques, Clark et al. (1987) published the "Detection of mycoplasma-related antigens in immune complexes from rheumatoid arthritis synovial fluids" in the Annals of Allergy.

What Constitutes Compelling Evidence?
Apparently our more detailed report on the "Antimycoplasma approach to the mechanism and control of rheumatoid disease," published in "Inflammatory Diseases and Copper" (Sorenson 1982), and described above, failed to provide NAAB with a level of compelling evidence. The report described the antibiotic treatment of spontaneous rheumatoid arthritis in gorilla models and a 5-year prospective study of 35 rheumatoid arthritis patients. As a result, both the NAAB panel of experts and NIH review questioned Brown's ability to diagnose rheumatoid arthritis, his knowledge of standard treatment, and his ability to measure clinical change.
Why did experts feel compelled to criticize the report and not investigate its merits?

The NIH critique of our report made it evident that we had to prove the benefits of tetracycline therapy to NIH before they would approve our grant request for support of a controlled clinical trial in order to provide the required compelling evidence. To support our claim, we hired an independent biostatistical firm to review Brown's hospitalized patients' records. The firm was certified by NIH so that the resulting data would be acceptable. To make the data as strong as possible, the firm was asked to review the charts of all patients Brown had hospitalized in the past 5 years (1978-1983) and select only those who they considered had rheumatoid arthritis. The firm even hired an independent rheumatologist, also approved by NIH, as a consultant to monitor the investigation and assure that the American Rheumatism Association's criteria for rheumatoid arthritis diagnosis were followed. The result was a retrospective study of 98 rheumatoid arthritis patients who began antibiotic (tetracycline) treatment during the 5-year

156

period. Their findings were reported at the 1985 International Rheumatology Congress in Sydney, Australia, by Brown and summarized as follows:

A Summary of the Independent Study Reported 1985.
An Independent Retrospective Analysis of Antibiotic therapy;
A study of 98 rheumatoid arthritis patients over 5 years

The biostatistical evaluations indicate that:

1. Eighty-four percent (84%) of the patients reported an improvement of 50% or more in their joints and in their morning stiffness. Seventy-five percent (75%) of the patients reported symptomatic improvement with respect to weakness, fatigue, depression and feeling of well being.

2. Sixty percent (60%) of the patients had previously received and subsequently discontinued gold therapy for reasons of insufficient response or toxicity prior to beginning antibiotic therapy. Many of the patients had also received other slow acting anti-rheumatic drugs which had been discontinued again for lack of effectiveness or toxicity.

3. Seventy percent (70%) of patients will remain on antibiotic therapy with continued control of their rheumatoid arthritis five years after starting treatment. By contrast other studies have shown that only 10 to 20 percent of patients treated with gold will remain on that drug for five years. What this means is that the chance of achieving a sustained improvement for five years from antibiotic treatment is as much as seven times better than with conventional gold therapy (see figure 1, p 158).

4. An unexpectedly positive and statistically significant correlation between duration of treatment and improvement was observed. In other words the patients continued to improve over the five year period of treatment, in contrast to the published reports on gold, penicillamine, and plaquenil, where improvement is not sustained (see figure 2, p159).

5. Patients on antibiotic therapy were able to reduce and in some cases discontinue their corticosteroid therapy, a critically important clinical observation.

6. No serious toxicities or side effects developed, in marked

157

contrast to the serious and sometimes life threatening side effects of gold, penicillamine or methotrexate.

In Summary:

The risks and benefits from the long term antibiotic treatment are substantially more favorable than the historical experience reported by other investigators using conventional slow acting drugs such as gold, penicillamine or plaquenil. Data from this retrospective five year study of 98 patients with definite or classical rheumatoid arthritis, who were treated with antibiotic therapy suggests better than expected outcomes based on current treatment standards.

Thus, antibiotic therapy appears to be associated with the-ability to maintain a majority of patients with rheumatoid arthritis in either a stable or an improved clinical state over a longer period of time with a lower degree of toxicity, with no serious side effects.

FIGURE 1. PROBABILITY OF RA PATIENTS REMAINING ON THERAPY

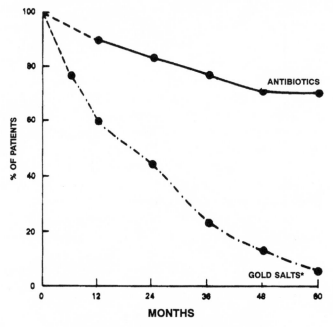

*CALCULATED FROM PUBLISHING DATA. (KEAN & ANASTASSIADES — 1979)

158

Publication of the completed study remains pending as the result of Brown's death. However, the completed manuscript was made available to NIH in hopes that the study would provide the compelling evidence to support a clinical trial of antibiotic therapy.

The results of the independent review of antibiotic therapy that were first briefly reported at the XVIth International Congress of Rheumatology in May 1985 received little attention except for a few rheumatologists who recognized the potential benefits. Reporters for *Medical World News* covered the meeting and prepared a special issue "The Arthritis—Infection Connection: Skeptics Reconsider." One of our pictures of a mycoplasma colony was used on the front cover with the article summarizing several reports on other possible infectious causes of rheumatoid arthritis. The article stated: "Excited doctors are on the verge of making one of the biggest break-throughs in the long search for a cure for the terrible agony of arthritis."

FIGURE 2. RHEUMATOID ARTHRITIS PATIENTS SUSTAINING 50% IMPROVEMENT ON LONG TERM TREATMENT

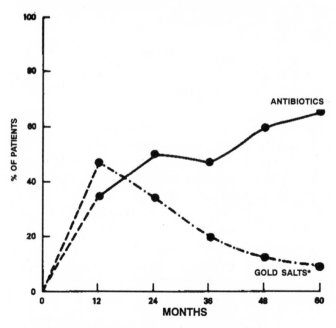

*CALCULATED FROM PUBLISHING DATA. (KEAN & ANASTASSIADES — 1979)

159

In 1951, 34 years prior to this report, newspaper and magazine headlines read "New Concept Reported Effective in Arthritis," when Brown et al. first reported and published in the *American Journal of Medical Science*, the early studies relating the control of rheumatoid arthritis by tetracycline's inhibition of the causative PPLO or mycoplasmas.

NIH Rejects Clinical Grant Applications

Backed by the independent evaluation of tetracycline therapy showing significant benefits for rheumatoid arthritis patients over a 5-year period, we submitted another grant application in June 1994 to NIH for the support of a multicenter controlled clinical trial to test the efficacy of tetracycline therapy. Even though no other 5-year study has shown the benefits of the approved therapies, the application was rejected, this time on technical grounds. The major reservation revolved around our proposal to use gold therapy as a positive control and not the more conventional ineffective placebo controls. Being convinced that tetracyclines would be much better than a blank placebo of aspirin, we decided to show that it was as good or better than gold, the approved drug of current choice, and thus limit additional trials.

Apparently the review committee's major concern was that without a placebo group on NSAIDS (aspirin) the study might not unequivocally determine whether this therapy works better than NSAIDS (antiinflammatory) drugs alone. Since most patients require at least the NSAID therapy, the test drug and placebo are usually given as a supplement. Although a double-blind controlled trial, including a placebo, is much more difficult and costly to conduct, with a higher dropout rate over an extended period, our institute agreed to revise and resubmit another application, including a placebo group as suggested. After spending thousands of precious research dollars and many more hours revising and reorganizing another multicenter trial, the second grant application was again rejected by the peer review committee. This time it was because there still was no compelling evidence to initiate a large and costly clinical trial of antibiotic therapy in rheumatic arthritis, as previously reported by the NAAB expert panel and NIH.

Usually our NIH grant applications for support of mycoplasma research have been approved but not funded because of limited research funds. Thus it seemed unusual that the clinical trial proposal was not approved for lack of sufficient funds. The lack of available funding by NIH perhaps was due in part to the 1985 establishment of the new National Institute of Arthritis and Musculoskeletal and Skin Diseases (NIAMSD), splitting off from NIADDK. What we and many others did not want was for Congress to establish another separate and costly bureaucratic institute that would usurp the already limited research funds. Thus as Congress later noted, there were less funds for research grants trying to find the cause and cure of the complex rheumatic diseases. In fact, two other NIH research grant applications that we submitted at that time to investigate the role of mycoplasma immune complexes in rheumatoid arthritis were approved but not funded. This seemed most unusual as the NIH clinical staff had recently reported that immune complexes and mycoplasmas were the top two probable causative factors.

What was more unusual and thought provoking was the remark by one of the rheumatologists on the NIH peer review committee, "What are you guys trying to do—put us out of business?" Yes, for the sake of 35 million arthritics, I certainly would like to close out a most costly business. Such remarks would seem to indicate that our supporting evidence was not only compelling but also threatening to their lucrative practices. In view of all the positive indicators, the experts' negative reactions made it difficult not to believe that they did not want our research team to find or even be recognized for finding a cure for rheumatoid arthritis.

Perhaps due in part to the emphasis placed on an infectious cause of rheumatoid arthritis at the International Rheumatism Congress in Australia and also our pursuit of the antimycoplasma approach to treatment, NIH held a 2-day workshop on "The Infectious Etiology of Early Arthritis" in November 1985 (as described above). The workshop probably was more motivated by the Congressional request for NIH to report to them on mycoplasma and antimycoplasma therapy in rheumatoid arthritis. This was acknowledged by the conference director, who recognized Brown for increasing the Congressional interest in this area, which included substantial appropriations for arthritis research. The thinking was that the infectious agent could best be detected and isolated as well as treated in the very early stages of rheumatoid arthritis as found in the animal models of mycoplasma arthritis. Although many reasonable recommendations were made concerning both basic research and clinical trials directed toward bacteria, mycoplasmas, and viruses, the workshop never got off the ground, as the director was unable to specify when, or if, and how much support would be available to implement the recommendations that were made. A prime example was not funding the two approved research grant applications that we had submitted. Actually, it was not the lack of NIH funds, as the new Arthritis Institute (NIAMSD) had over $100,000,000 in appropriations to support arthritis-related research.

Priorities for Antimycoplasma Treatment
In its 1987 appropriations of $140,225,000 for NIAMSD, Congress reported that "A growing body of evidence implicates microorganisms, bacteria, mycoplasma, and viruses, and the prevailing theory is that one or more of these organisms precipitate immune responses that induce arthritis signs and symptoms in genetically predisposed persons. Research studies are seeking to discern the role of infectious agents in early arthritis." The Appropriations Committee usually reports on what the NIH directors ask it to support. Other testimony at the budget hearings included, "For the past few years, the committee has heard testimony in support of the positive results of antibiotic treatment for rheumatoid arthritis. Testimony has been presented to the committee which indicates that mycoplasmas may be one of the infectious causes of rheumatoid disease. The committee suggests that the NIH continue to monitor the research underway and give full consideration to support a prospective controlled clinical trial of antibiotic therapy for rheumatoid arthritis."

Apparently when the Congressional committee reviewed our favorable report on the 5-year antibiotic treatment of 98 patients with rheumatoid arthritis and the rationale behind our rejected multi-center grant application, they decided, contrary to the NAAB and NIH recommendations, that there was sufficient and compelling evidence to warrant a large clinical trial. Nearly 3 years later (April 1989), 2 weeks after Brown's death, NIAMSD finally took

162

action and requested proposals from clinical centers for grant applications to assess the efficacy of minocycline in rheumatoid arthritis. At long last, 40 years after a trial was first proposed in 1949 by Brown, NIH began seeking applicants to serve as clinical centers for a randomized, double-blind, placebo-controlled trial that would assess the efficacy of tetracycline in the treatment of rheumatoid arthritis.

Mycoplasmas are one of the few suspected causes of rheumatoid arthritis even though the supporting evidence still remains insufficient to some. Like the origin of the currently approved gold therapy that was directed toward the unknown but suspected Tb cause, therapy could and should be directed toward the elimination of a suspected cause, especially if the proposed therapy is safer and less costly. Similarly, other clinical trials should also be directed toward the other suspected bacterial or viral causes to determine which therapy is most effective, even though the infectious cause remains unknown. Such therapeutic probes would at least put us closer to the target that must be reached if the permanent cure and prevention is to be achieved.

NIH Protocol for a Minocycline Clinical Trial
NIH-supported clinical trial of tetracycline's effectiveness in rheumatoid arthritis patients, which was requested by Congress, is described in their Protocol and Patient Management called "Minocycline in Rheumatoid Arthritis (MIRA)." In brief, the clinical trial includes:

Objective:
To determine whether minocycline hydrochloride produces meaningful improvement (defined as a net 50% improvement in the joint counts for tender and swollen joints) in patients with rheumatoid arthritis.

To determine the frequency and severity of adverse effects of minocycline-HCl in patients with rheumatoid arthritis.

Overview:
The objectives of this collaborative (multi-center) clinical trial can be met randomizing (200) volunteer rheumatoid arthritis

patients within the clinical centers into an actively treated group that would receive two capsules containing 50 mg. of minocycline-HCl twice a day and a control group that would receive physically indistinguishable placebo capsules between meals on an empty stomach continuously for 48 weeks.

Study medication may be reduced or temporarily discontinued if toxicity ensues. After toxicity abates the medication may then be either restarted and/or increased to the maximum tolerated dose (up to 200 mg. per day).

Medication Restrictions:

1. If on NSAIDS or aspirin, patients can remain on the stable dose. If not—cannot be started.

2. If on Prednisone, 10 mg/day maximum, must remain constant.

3. Patients will have been off DMARDs and injectable steroids 4 weeks.

Selection and Exclusion of Patients:

The inclusion of volunteer patients in the clinical trial is highly selective together with close monthly monitoring that includes blood tests and quarterly assessments. The patient recruiting started in 1991 and the results are expected to be reported in 1993 or 1994, depending on when the 200th and last volunteer patient is accepted.

* * *

After 40 plus years trying to get NIH and the medical community to test tetracycline's effectiveness in rheumatoid arthritis patients, it was great to see the clinical trial finally started. Of course it would have been more enjoyable if we could have participated and shared in the recognition. The protocol introduction stated: "It has been proposed that rheumatoid arthritis may have an infectious etiology; possible agents include viruses and bacteria such as mycoplasma. However, despite intensive efforts, no infectious agent has been isolated. Nonetheless, some rheumatologists have long advocated tetracycline antibiotics as an appropriate treatment for rheumatoid arthritis (Brown, et al, 1959, Sanchez, 1968)." This one reference to Brown's lifelong work was a 32-page chapter in the medical textbook on *Long Term Illness*, discussing the "Management of the Chronically Ill Patient." Many other references to his reports in 1949 and 1951 and our more recent reports in 1982 and 1988, would have provided the clinicians more perspective and information on the subject.

Strangely enough, the completed minocycline clinical trial did not look or test for any of the suspected infectious agents. Why did NIH fail to look for antibodies to infectious agents, especially when rheumatoid arthritis is suspected to be an immunologic response to some infectious agent or its immune complex? Any benefits obtained from the high daily doses of minocycline (200 mg/day), inhibiting the destructive collagenase enzyme and any infectious agent (such as mycoplasma), may be outweighed by tetracycline's tissue toxicity unless administered in the pulsed intermittent doses (alternating days) that we have recommended. Unless the clinicians realize that they are treating an immunologic disorder and not an infectious disease with a potent chelating agent, the full therapeutic benefits may not be achieved. In fact, the investigators may now blindly go the other way and try to develop another more potent anti-inflammatory or anticollagenase symptomatic drug. Fortunately, Congress has requested NIH to conduct 5-year trials of both oral and intravenous tetracycline therapy and also monitor the rheumatoid arthritis patients for mycoplasma antibodies, which would help to focus on the infectious cause.

As mentioned above, on November 8, 1993, the participating six American clinics briefly reported the results of their 48-week double-blind trial of minocycline at the national meeting of the American College of Rheumatology. They reported the minocycline to be beneficial and safe in the rheumatoid arthritis patients treated. Publication of the detailed results in a medical journal for all doctors to evaluate should provide the long-awaited confirmation.

At the same meeting and in essential agreement with the American trial, a group in the Netherlands and one in Israel also reported that minocycline is beneficial in rheumatoid arthritis patients and relatively safe even when given with other medications.

As a background in the press release for the news media, the American College of Rheumatology stated: "In 1988, researcher

Thomas McPherson Brown, M.D., presented a study showing that minocycline was effective in the treatment of rheumatoid arthritis. Most researchers felt that the methods used to conduct the study were not adequate to support the claims. Dr. Brown died before he could conduct further research." One year prior to his death, Brown published his book *The Road Back: Rheumatoid Arthritis—Its Cause and Its Treatment* (Evans 1988),which discusses many of his earlier studies and publications over the past 50 years. He reported the first successful treatment of rheumatoid arthritis patients with tetracycline in 1949 at the national rheumatology meeting when the curative benefits of cortisone were promoted. Although the methods he used 40 years ago may not seem adequate today, the rationale for such studies in preference to cortisone is stronger than ever.

Rationale for Antimycoplasma Treatment

1. Tetracyclines and other related antibiotics are used in the treatment of mycoplasma infections.

2. Mycoplasmas are known or suspected to cause arthritis in many different animals, including gorillas, elephants, and humans.

3. Gold salts first used to empirically treat arthritis in humans also inhibits mycoplasma growth and controls arthritis in animals infected with mycoplasmas.

4. Parenteral (injected) tetracyclines were found to be more effective than oral in controlling mycoplasma infection in arthritic animals and humans.

5. Because of the toxicity and side effects of gold, plaquenil, and penicillamine treatment, zoo veterinarians have had to use tetracycline as a safe alternative to successfully treat their valuable and precious arthritic animals, especially those testing mycoplasma positive.

6. Mycoplasmas can cause a variety of diseases in animals and humans, including arthritis and other symptoms related to rheumatoid disorders.

7. The persistence and low cytopathogenicity of the ubiquitous mycoplasmas makes them a probable cause of chronic rheumatoid arthritis in humans.

166

8. Mycoplasmas that strongly adhere to tissue cells are more difficult to isolate and identify in and eliminate from the human host. Routine oral antibiotic therapy does not always eliminate mycoplasmas or their antibodies.

9. Doctors not knowing the infectious cause of rheumatoid arthritis should test patients for possible mycoplasma and other infections by culture or serology. Patients testing positive should be treated with antibiotic therapy, especially if they have failed on the symptomatic therapy.

10. Rheumatoid arthritis patients testing serologically positive for mycoplasmas should be diagnosed as arthritis complicated with mycoplasmas and treated with appropriate antimycoplasma medications.

Mycoplasmas, in addition to their immunopathogenic role as an autoantigen carrier and immune complex components, can attach firmly to receptive tissue cell sites, especially the blood vessels and nerves, where they could interfere with cellular functions. These reactive disease mechanisms are the result of mycoplasmas' unusual characteristics. Not having a cell wall and unlike bacteria and viruses, mycoplasmas are contained in a bilayered proteolipid membrane that binds to many different cell surfaces (including glass). Mycoplasmas also selectively bind specific basic cellular proteins (gamma globulins and myelin basic proteins) and thus acquire and promote non-self properties of their cellular components. In addition, mycoplasmas, like animals but unlike bacteria and viruses, require cholesterol for growth; and like humans, the higher the cholesterol content of their growth media the higher their cholesterol composition. As a result, mycoplasmas growing in a human with a high blood cholesterol level will in turn also have a high cholesterol content. Only in this case, mycoplasmas do not have coronary heart disease but could cause it, or atherosclerosis, by depositing their cholesterol-loaded cells in the coronary arteries and elsewhere. Other pathogenic mechanisms may be identified in the near future when mycoplasma's fingerprints (DNA) are detected in the brain and neural plaques of Alzheimer's and multiple sclerosis patients as well as in arterial plaques. Even though mycoplasmas have a special affinity for the basic mucoproteins in the joint tissues and blood vessels, there is every reason to believe that they can and will be found in many other tissues associated with other chronic immunologic disorders, such as diabetes.

American Rheumatism Association's Views
The American Rheumatism Association, now the American College of Rheumatology, is the world's largest professional organization of physicians and scientists dedicated to providing leadership in rheumatology research, education, and patient care and thus is responsible for finding the cause and cures of rheumatoid disorders.

In 1988, Dr. Brown's book began to receive media attention. The president of the American Rheumatism Association, with help from the Arthritis Foundation, issued a letter and position paper or fact sheet to its members and associates in order to help them respond to any inquires about the book. In his letter, the president stated that "Dr. Brown has indicated that there is a demonstrated relationship between infection with mycoplasma and the development of rheumatoid arthritis. He also concludes that antibiotic therapy, specifically tetracycline, is effective therapy or even a cure for rheumatoid arthritis. The ARA agrees completely with the NAAB report, cited above, that they could not find any 'sound' evidence for a relationship between mycoplasma infection and the development of rheumatoid arthritis, and from data presently available (April 1988), antibiotic therapy has not been proven to be effective therapy for rheumatoid arthritis."

Chapter X
Rheumatoid Arthritis—
Causes and Treatment

The following is the American Rheumatism Association's fact sheet with the author's comments in brackets:

The cause of rheumatoid arthritis is unknown and there is presently no known cure. However, rheumatologists, who provide specialized medical care for people with arthritis, have established many effective treatments for rheumatoid arthritis.

[Many patients and doctors would contest this claim.]

Infection may play a role in causing rheumatoid arthritis:

• Epstein Barr (EB) virus and parvovirus, as well as several other viruses, have been suggested to play a role in some people with the disease. *[If so, why not test anti-viral therapy?]*

• Lyme arthritis, which resembles rheumatoid arthritis, was discovered to be caused by a type of bacteria known as a spirochete.

[Which is not rheumatoid arthritis but is best treated with intravenous tetracycline.]

• Through carefully designed research, other agents may be found to play a role in causing rheumatoid arthritis. *[Such as what? When and who will carefully design the research to find the causes of rheumatoid arthritis? If the patients benefit from tetracycline therapy, it does not matter what agents are playing a role.]*

- Extensive investigations to date have not produced any convincing scientific evidence that mycoplasma plays a role in causing rheumatoid arthritis.

[Some people are harder to convince. Why not at least try tetracycline therapy? The American Rheumatism Association has been promoting the use of toxic antimalarial therapy for years and never proved malaria was the cause of rheumatoid arthritis.]

- Modern techniques of molecular biology are available which can now determine whether or not a specific infectious agent is present in a person.

[Why haven't these modern techniques been used? We have, and found mycoplasmas.]

- The American Rheumatism Association strongly supports further sound, scientific research in this area.

[When, where, or what? Recent reports from around the world all seem to favor tetracycline therapy.]

Other factors are believed to be involved in the cause of rheumatoid arthritis:

- The rapidly emerging field of molecular genetics is shedding important new light on the genetic susceptibility of some people to develop rheumatoid arthritis.

[A patient's genetic susceptibility is not the primary cause nor the solution.]

- The immune system is known to be involved in the development of rheumatoid arthritis and new clues are rapidly accumulating about its role.

[The immune system responds to the foreign antigen or infectious cause. Many factors are involved in the resulting symptoms or host reactions.]

170

The National Institutes of Health and the National Arthritis Advisory Board appointed a panel of experts in the field of rheumatology to examine the hypothesis that mycoplasma is a cause of rheumatoid arthritis. The American Rheumatism Association fully supports the following conclusions of the 1983 report of the panel. *[The panel members are also members of the association and certainly are not impartial. Apparently and fortunately, the U.S. Congress does not support their conclusions.]*

- Dr. Brown has implied that the sequence of infection with mycoplasma through to development of rheumatic arthritis has been demonstrated in man. It certainly has not. It is possible that mycoplasma could cause rheumatoid arthritis but there are no direct confirmations of this hypothesis.
[If it is possible, why hasn't the association attempted to prove or disprove the mycoplasma cause or the benefits of antimycoplasma tetracycline therapy?]

- Reports of antimycoplasma agents (e.g., tetracycline) being efficacious in treatment of rheumatoid arthritis are not documented by objective criteria and are not sufficient to warrant a broad-scale study of these drugs in rheumatoid arthritis. In particular the panel recommended strongly against any study done without double-blind controls in a randomized trial. The placebo effect of skilled, confident and compassionate deliverers of health care can never be underestimated.
[If mycoplasmas are a possible cause, why hasn't the association leadership tested and provided the objective criteria? Why hasn't it reviewed the patients' charts that document the efficacy of tetracycline treatment rather than just parrot the NIH report?]

- The only logical approach to conducting any treatment trial would be a prospective, controlled double-blind study involving people who were found to have evidence of mycoplasma infection in their joints.
[This recommendation (also made by NIH) is an illogical and unethical approach in a misguided attempt to test for the mycoplasma cause but certainly not the therapeutic effectiveness. Mycoplasma infectious

171

arthritis in the joints is not necessarily rheumatoid arthritis but is treated with intraarticular tetracycline.]

• There has been no publication of the results of tetracycline therapy in rheumatoid arthritis by Dr. Brown and his colleagues in which parameters of disease activity are measured in double-blind fashion. A 1971 study by Skinner, et al. (Arthritis and Rheumatism, 14: 727, 1971), using doses of tetracycline previously reported by Brown et al. to be effective therapy of rheumatoid arthritis, was a double-blind study for one year. There was no difference in the course of treated compared with control patients. *[See the positive minocycline results recently reported (1993) by the American College of Rheumatology. Which trial do they now believe? Apparently Brown and his colleagues were right on target and should have been supported rather than criticized as unproven quackery.]*

• The great majority of patients with rheumatoid arthritis respond satisfactorily to regimens of proven efficacy. Such treatments include a wide range of nonsteroidal anti-inflammatory drugs and other medications capable of modifying the course of the disease and, for some individuals, putting the disease in remission. Treatment also includes physical and occupational therapy, including programs of exercise. The dangers in the use of unproven remedies are that those of known effectiveness may be overlooked or neglected.
[Where are the long-term double-blind criteria on the proven remedies that are now being recognized as nonmodifying failures? The costly double-blind trials did not predict the present drug failures.]

* * *

Who should the 30 plus million arthritic patients believe? What are the facts when the American Rheumatism Association says the proven treatment is satisfactory for a great majority of patients while the doctors at NIH are concerned that the treatment is very unsatisfactory. Only the patients know the truth. The author will leave it up to the patients who read *The Road Back* to decide whether the criticism leveled against Brown's work by the American Rheumatism Association was really beneficial and showed their leadership role.

172

Promising Therapies for Rheumatoid Diseases

Although the Arthritis Foundation's publication *Arthritis Today* (February 1990) failed to mention tetracycline in its article "Promising Therapies of The 90's: Arthritis Research Enters a New Decade," it was mentioned later in the December 1990 issue. In the question and answer section, a patient asked: "I have been advised by my physician to take tetracycline to help cure rheumatoid arthritis. Is this treatment safe and successful or just another false hope for rheumatoid arthritis sufferers?" The Arthritis Foundation's answer was: "Although tetracycline has been shown to influence the composition of certain tissues grown in a laboratory setting, it has not been established as an effective treatment for rheumatoid arthritis. A large and carefully controlled study of tetracycline in the treatment of rheumatoid arthritis has not been done, although one is now being undertaken by the NIAMSD."

[The question remains unanswered why the Arthritis Foundation did not list tetracycline as a promising therapy and when they will tell patients about the beneficial results of tetracycline treatment recently reported by the NIH supported clinics.]

I seriously doubt that NIH would conduct this costly controlled trial if it did not consider tetracycline therapy promising with compelling reasons, such as the Congressional Appropriations Committee. Knowing that NIH had undertaken a very costly (over $4 million) tetracycline clinical trial, it seems unusual that tetracyclines were not mentioned as one of the promising therapies of the 1990s.

Since the article's information came directly from NIH, citing both new and old medications, the therapeutic benefits were all downgraded as "There is no quick fix for arthritis and no one can say when or if a specific treatment will be available." Scientists keep reporting that the outlook for arthritis is bright, while patients keep asking whether doctors will ever find a way to stop their disease. From what has appeared in the medical literature over the past 20 years, the arthritis patients' future is not very bright unless the clinical research and treatment are redirected toward eliminating probable infectious causes and not just the resulting symptoms. Except for the tetracycline antibiotics, the so-called promising therapies seem to offer the same misguided future.

Perhaps the darkest cloud hanging over the rheumatoid patients' heads is the current desperate pursuit of combination chemotherapy. When three of the most toxic and dangerous drugs are being investigated by NIH as the most promising cure for rheumatoid arthritis, the patients should scream "Why?" Billions of patients' tax dollars are going to support arthritis research that has yet to come up with a satisfactory and long-lasting disease-modifying therapy. These patients are further penalized when they also pay dearly for costly tests and ineffective and toxic therapy. This is why patients are finally asking Congress to tell NIH what direction to pursue.

Patients Push Congress

For years, arthritis patients have been trying to get their doctors to try the tetracycline therapy that has been labeled unproven and experimental by the establishment. Some doctors strongly objected when their patients requested tetracycline, while others secretly gave the antibiotic. When only a few doctors dared to step forward to give tetracycline a trial, the arthritis patients, who were tired of living with their disease and sick of being told for the past 40 years that the cause and cure were unknown, took their problem to Congress and requested help. With over $200 million a year appropriated for NIAMSD, the taxpaying patients have a good reason to ask why a cure or cause has not been found. Every year, Congress appropriates additional millions more for arthritis research that only has resulted in greater costs to the patients for diagnostic tests and stopgap treatment as the approved disease-modifying therapies become ineffective, more costly, and dangerous.

In the 1993 budget of $214 million for NIAMSD, the Appropriations Committee made several requests and recommendations aimed at finding the long sought answers to the perpetuated rheumatoid disease problems.

"The committee is concerned that the proportion of funds to support initiatives in arthritis research have not kept pace with the overall growth of the Institute. When the new Arthritis Institute, NIAMSD, was established (in 1985) arthritis and related musculoskeletal disease research comprised 50% of the Institute's budget, whereas in the 1993 budget request only 38% of the Insti-

174

tute's budget is directed toward research in this area.

"The committee is pleased that promising advances are being made in understanding mechanisms of joint destruction, control of the inflammatory process, and genetics of this disease that affects over 2 million Americans. In a major clinical trial, the drug minocycline is being evaluated for efficacy and safety. Results of the trial, conducted at six clinical sites, are expected in the spring of 1994, and may provide a new treatment for rheumatoid arthritis. This trial now has been completed and reported as beneficial and safe, while the patients still wait for action. "Within the funds provided, at least $3,000,000 is earmarked for mycoplasma research pertaining to rheumatoid arthritis and other rheumatic diseases with special emphasis on initiating clinical trials on the intravenous antibiotic treatment of rheumatoid arthritis and other rheumatic diseases. The clinical trials should monitor mycoplasma antibody levels present in the patients."

The Ten Year NIH Report (1982-1992)
Bernadine Healy, M.D., Director, NIH and
Lawrence E. Shulman, M.D., Ph.D.

As for background, a five page Ten Year Report dated January 1993, submitted by the director of the National Institutes of Health [NIH] in response to the Senate's request was entitled "Mycoplasma Research, Infectious Disease Theory Research, or Antibiotic Clinical Trials." Portions of the Ten Year Report are included here.

"In 1982, the Committee [on appropriations] included the following report language: 'The Committee wishes to be kept apprised of the Institute's [NIH] research into mycoplasma-related causes of rheumatoid arthritis. The Committee expects the Institute to examine relevant clinical data and report back within a year its assessment of whatever line of inquiry may be suggested. Such a review should take into account the possible importance of duration of treatment as a variable in evaluating the mycoplasma perspective. The report prepared in response to that request contained specific recommendations as to the research approach to be followed. Since 10 years have elapsed since the preparation of that report the Committee would like an assessment of the progress made by the Institute in implementing these recommendations. The Committee would like to have a report by February 1, 1993, detailing the amounts of awards of grants for either mycoplasma research, infectious disease theory research, or antibiotic clinical trials before and after 1982" (Senate Report 102-397, page 126).

The Ten Year Report report cited the previous two NIH reports in 1983 and 1984 (discussed above) that were requested by the House and Senate Appropriations Committees on mycoplasma, infectious theory research, and antibiotic treatment and their relationship to rheumatoid arthritis. In addition, NIH submitted a third report entitled "Report on Antibiotic therapy for Rheumatoid Arthritis: Clinical Trials and Related Research" (Senate Report No. 98-544). More recently, a NIH report entitled "Clinical Trial to Assess the Efficacy of Minocycline in the Treatment of Rheumatoid Arthritis and Mycoplasma Research" was prepared in response to a request contained in Senate Report No. 101-516 for FY 1991, which introduced the MIRA clinical trial described above.

[Although the 10-year report listed the total annual amounts awarded each year for infectious arthritis research as requested, there was little mention of the accomplishments or progress made toward finding the infectious causes or the cure for rheumatoid arthritis.]

This latest Ten Year NIH report summarized and paraphrased their previous recommendations made ten years ago:

1. "Insufficient evidence existed in 1983 to warrant a large-scale, costly, clinical trial of antimycoplasma therapy for rheumatoid arthritis.

2. "Research using mycoplasma-induced arthritis in animals as models for rheumatoid arthritis in humans was useful and should continue.

3. "The NAAB panel of experts recommended a two-stepped, sequential approach for evaluating the role of antimycoplasma therapy consisting of:

    a. Collection of samples of synovial fluid and tissue from 100 patients with rheumatoid arthritis and 100 patients with nonrheumatoid arthritis for analysis by at least two laboratories for evidence of mycoplasma. chronic arthritis for analysis by at least two laboratories for evidence of mycoplasma.

b. If positive results were obtained, a double-blind controlled clinical trial of long-term antimycoplasma therapy should be considered in patients demonstrated to be culture- or antigen-positive for mycoplasma."

[The 10-year NIH report seems to be saying that there was insufficient evidence and funds to conduct our proposed clinical trial of tetracycline, but it was okay for NIH to conduct even more costly, questionable, and untested procedures. And what is even more ironical is that NIH was completing a large clinical trial of minocycline that was found to be beneficial and safe in rheumatoid arthritis patients.]

Progress Toward Implementing the Recommendations

The report further states that NIH did not initiate the clinical trial of antimycoplasma therapy for rheumatoid arthritis although the trial had been recommended by the NIH and the NAAB expert panel. However, the 1984 NIH report described their efforts to "support a clinical trial of antibiotic therapy for rheumatoid arthritis and developments from related research that provided a scientific foundation for such a clinical trial and new information about the actions of minocycline, an antiobiotic from the tetracycline family."

The report goes on to say, "During 1983, the National Institute of Arthritis, Diabetes, and Digestive and Kidney Diseases (NIADDK), actively worked with Dr. Thomas McPherson Brown, Dr. Howard (sic) W. Clarke and their colleagues at the Arthritis Institute of the National Hospital in Arlington, Virginia, who were applying for research grant support for a clinical trial to assess the efficacy of tetracycline treatment of rheumatoid arthritis. They were unsuccessful in obtaining grant support.

"At about the same time [1983], developments from dental research were providing insights into an alternative mechanism of action that might explain the perceived benefit of minocycline in the treatment of rheumatoid arthritis, other than its antibiotic action against mycoplasma or other infectious agents. Researchers had found that, independent of its antimicrobial properties, minocycline inhibited the action of a tissue-destroying enzyme (collagenase) released by inflamed tissues in diabetic rats with periodontal disease. Collagenase is also released by inflamed joints in rheuma-

toid arthritis, contributing to joint damage.
[This inhibiting action of tetracyclines had been known for many years, but what causes the tissue inflammation that activates the collagenase?]

"Encouraged by these results, clinical researchers investigated the effects of giving minocycline orally to patients with rheumatoid arthritis for ten days prior to joint surgery. They found that this resulted in reduced levels of collagenase in synovial tissue and fluid in patients receiving minocycline.
[Orthopedic surgeons at the National Hospital for Orthopedics and Rehabilitation had frequently observed a better response to surgery in Brown's tetracycline-treated patients, with less inflammation and faster healing.]

The report continues, "In addition, minocycline and the other tetracyclines have been found to have other biologic effects that might be beneficial in treating rheumatoid arthritis such as their immunosuppressive and immunomodulating properties. Using two widely accepted animal models of rheumatoid arthritis (type II collagen and adjuvant arthritis in rats) researchers, supported by the National Institute of Arthritis and Musculoskeletal and Skin Diseases, (NIAMS), found that adding minocycline to the drinking water impaired the production and metabolism of inflammatory cells important in the pathogenesis of arthritis in these animals.
[The pertinent question is why the researchers did not test the more natural mycoplasma-induced arthritis animal models that are supported by NIH grants.]

"Based on these new leads, the NIAMS proceeded with soliciting a research contract proposals (two weeks after Dr. Brown was lost to cancer in 1989) for six clinical centers and a coordinating center to conduct what is now called the Minocycline in Rheumatoid Arthritis (MIRA) Trial. The planning phase for MIRA, during which the final protocol and related study documents were developed, began in April 1991 and was completed that October. Accrual of patient [volunteers] began in November 1991 and was completed in May 1992 after 219 patients had been enrolled and

178

randomized to minocyline or placebo treatment.

[NIH has taken over 40 years (1949-1991) to finally recognize and support the merits of tetracycline in rheumatoid arthritis that Brown developed and first introduced, which finally warranted the Senate's persuasive push. The compelling evidence that NIH demanded from us before supporting a clinical trial apparently was not found in the thousands of rheumatoid patients Brown had successfully treated and tested for mycoplasmas over the past 40 years. Coincidentally, NIH found sufficient evidence for a clinical trial only after the Appropriations Committee had requested them to conduct a trial. This was shortly after the American Rheumatism Association (1988) had concurred with NIH that the objective criteria for tetracycline therapy was not sufficient to warrant a broad scale study.]

"The MIRA protocol calls for 48 weeks of active treatment [200mg/day]; therefore, the results of the trial will be available in 1993 in time, it is hoped, for presentation at the American College of Rheumatology annual scientific meeting in November 1993. Final results will be available for reporting to the Appropriations Committees during the hearings on the Fiscal Year 1995 budget in the Spring of 1994. The results will be widely disseminated through publication in a peer-reviewed journal as well.

[If the publication of the beneficial results of the MIRA trial is found to be safe and effective, who will get the credit and what is NIH going to advise the patients and doctors? The 30 million tax-paying arthritics will want to know why they have had to suffer 40 years waiting for NIH to launch an investigation of tetracycline therapy.]

The Ten Year Report Continues:
The Institute has continued to support research on mycoplasma-induced arthritis in animal models of rheumatoid arthritis in humans. The amounts of awards of grants for mycoplasma research supported by the NIADDK (Fiscal years 1981 through 1985) and subsequently by the NIAMS (Fiscal years 1986 through 1992)totaled $3.4 million dollars.

[If NIH was supporting so much for mycoplasma research in models of rheumatoid arthritis, why were our reports in 1981, 1985, 1989 at the International Rheumatology Congresses the only papers on mycoplas-

mas in rheumatoid arthritis? Why weren't there any reports on myco-
plasma in rheumatoid arthritis presented at the 1992 and the 1994
International Mycoplasmology meetings? Of the reported $31.4 mil-
lion funded for infectious arthritis Research during the past 6 years
(1987-1992) 5% or $1.5 million went to support mycoplasma induced
arthritis. I seriously doubt that arthritis patients would consider spend-
ing only 0.2% of the total 1992 appropriations to find the cause and
cure of arthritis "taking the mycoplasma cause of rheumatoid arthri-
tis seriously", as NIH previously reported.]

"Mycoplasmas are not the only infectious agents that have
been implicated as etiologic agents or triggers for arthritis. Other
infectious agents of interest include the Epstein Barr virus, various
retroviruses and the DNA parvoviruses; Klebsiella, Yersinia, Chlamy-
dia, Shigella and Salmonella bacteria; and Borrelia burgdorferi, the
spirochete that causes Lyme disease. Support by the NIAMS for all
aspects of infectious arthritis research has increased greatly since
the [new] Institute was created. The funding for infectious arthritis by the NIAMS has been $31.4 million dollars (fiscal years 1987
through 1992).

[Where are the results from animal models of these other infectious
agents? Where are the antibiotic or antiviral clinical trials? Over 20
years ago, (1972), NIH reported to the Senate committee that myco-
plasma-induced arthritis in pigs was the perfect model of rheumatoid
arthritis and would be pursued. Where are the results? The NIH in-
vestigators also found what we had previously reported—that the myco-
plasma antibodies persisted in the gorilla model as well as the
rheumatoid patients when mycoplasmas were no longer isolated. The
Appropriations Committee has now requested NIH to monitor myco-
plasma antibody levels in patients in association with intravenous tet-
racycline therapy. Has NIH supported any projects that monitored
antibody levels to the other suspected infectious agents in rheumatoid
patients? It should be noted that the acute infectious (septic) arthritis
in animals is not chronic rheumatoid arthritis.]

The Ten Year Report further stated, "NIADDK took some
initial steps toward implementing the recommendation of the NAAB
for a two-stepped, sequential approach for evaluating antimyco-

180

plasma therapy; however, the developments from dental research described above motivated the Institute (NIH) to pursue the initiation of the MIRA Trial directly . . . . The seven research contracts to accomplish this trial were negotiated and awarded in 1991. By the time of its completion the MIRA trial will have cost slightly more than four million dollars.

[Apparently the MIRA trial was not budgeted under Infectious Agents. The clinical trial we proposed 6 years earlier but not approved by NIH was budgeted for half as much, $2,000,000. The question remains, what are NIH, the Arthritis Foundation, and the American Rheumatism Association going to advise the doctors and patients when they are now told that tetracycline therapy has been proven safe and effective. What is their next step?]

The Ten Year progress report by NIH also included their future plans: Fiscal Year 1993 Research Institutes.

"By early 1993, the NIAMSD will have issued a Request for Applications (RFA) for research investigating the relationship between mycoplasma and other infectious agents and chronic systemic rheumatic diseases. This RFA will be issued in collaboration with the National Institute of Allergy and Infectious Diseases which also has an interest in this line of research. The goal of the RFA will be to stimulate research into whether any of the chronic inflammatory rheumatic diseases might be caused by infection, and if so, which infection and by what mechanisms."

[What infectious cause or antibiotic cure of any of the other 99 rheumatic diseases has NIH supported in the past 10 years with their billion dollars of appropriations? Did NIH support (1982-1992) any grants looking for the infectious cause or tetracycline cure in Juvenile Rheumatoid Arthritis, Lupus, scleroderma, or any of the other rheumatic diseases? Why hasn't NIH supported research on the infectious cause and the minocycline treatment of other chronic inflammatory disorders? Finally recognizing tetracycline's anti-inflammatory and immunosuppressive properties, how many grants were awarded to test its effectiveness in other inflammatory immunologic or autoimmune disorders? Is NIH again waiting for the diabetes and multiple sclerosis patients to tell Congress where and what NIH should be researching? Why has it taken NIH 17 years to pursue actions recommended

in the master Arthritis Plan of 1976?]

<u>Conclusions of the Ten Year Report</u>
"The NIAMSD has continued to support and encourage research related to infectious causes of arthritis, including mycoplasmas. The new RFA will stimulate additional research to address these important questions. The Institute (NIH) has implemented a double-blind, placebo-controlled clinical trial of minocycline therapy for rheumatoid arthritis. The results from this clinical trial should answer many questions about the safety and efficacy of long-term administration of [oral] minocycline to patients with rheumatoid arthritis.

[Yes, but what is the infectious cause of rheumatoid arthritis or any one of the other rheumatoid diseases that could provide leads to its cure and prevention? For a few more dollars, why not include tests for mycoplasma antibody levels, as Congress suggested. What about other antibiotic clinical trials for longer periods and the intermittent or intravenous treatment that Congress requested? Many questions proposed 40 years ago still remain unanswered.]

* * *

The measure of accomplishment apparently is not how much has been awarded for research grants in the past 10 years, but how much has been discovered about the cause and the cure of rheumatoid diseases? Many grants have been awarded for mycoplasma research, but how much of that was directed toward finding the causes of human diseases? How much has been learned about a safer and more effective therapy? In the past 10 years, NIAMSD has been appropriated over one billion tax dollars for arthritis and related disorders. What new causes or new cures have been discovered? With countless billions more also being spent for ineffective palliative therapy, as well as on unproven remedies, everyone seems to be benefitting and getting richer except the arthritis patients and their families. Being the most crippling, most prevalent, and most costly to treat, especially in medical disability payments, Congress and the patients should demand greater than the 0.2 percent research effort to find answers to these complex rheumatic diseases. The

182

patients should also ask the Arthritis Foundation and the American College of Rheumatology, the so-called leaders responsible for finding the answer to arthritis.

CHAPTER XI
A Bright, Arthritis-Free Future

Now at long last, having learned to live with rheumatoid disorders, it looks like something is being done to reduce, if not eliminate, these major medical, economic, and social burdens. Thanks to Congressional concerns, the Appropriations Committee in their 1990 budget for NIH stated the need to pursue both the clinical trials of tetracycline therapy and the investigation of the role of mycoplasmas in rheumatoid diseases. In the 1993 NIH budget, at least $3,000,000 was earmarked by the committee for mycoplasma research pertaining to rheumatoid arthritis and other diseases. The committee also said that special emphasis should be placed on initiating clinical trials on the intravenous antibiotic treatment of rheumatoid arthritis and other rheumatic diseases. The clinical trials should also monitor mycoplasma antibody levels present in the patients. Our laboratory had been monitoring mycoplasma antibody levels in the antibiotic-treated rheumatoid arthritis patients, as well as gorillas and elephants, for over 20 years. Brown et al. had been treating rheumatoid arthritis patients successfully with intravenous antibiotics for over 40 years, as they had first reported in 1951 (Am. J. Med. Sci. 221: 1951) which resulted in newspaper headlines around the world. What happened to that news story on the rheumatic disease breakthrough? How and why did it get buried?

Now 43 years later, with clinical trials supported by NIH, there should be no question of direction since the door has finally been opened and confirmation is available. Along with NIH, the medical community should now give mycoplasmas another special look and try both oral and intravenous tetracycline therapy in the other inflammatory rheumatoid collagen vascular diseases, also called chronic infectious arthritis. At that time, the new therapy was heralded in a special publication by *Newsweek,* and *Popular Science* (December, 1951) described the research as one of the "10 Biggest Science Stories of 1951." As one science writer reported (1952) in *Life Today,* "Never has the outlook for arthritis been as promising as at present. As time goes on and as the extensive research which is now being conducted sheds further light on this elusive ailment, patients may look ahead to a time when they may be free of their affliction rather than having their disease merely arrested."

The new findings and concept on the cause and treatment were presented by Brown's assistant, Ruth H. Wichelhausen, director of the VA hospital's rheumatic disease research, at the national meeting of the American Rheumatic Association in Atlantic City, New Jersey, on June 8, 1951. The paper was simultaneously published in the *American Journal of Medical Sciences.* The preliminary report had been presented at the October, 1950 meeting of the American Clinical and Climatological Association.

In response to his grant application and the 1951 report on the antibiotic treatment of rheumatoid arthritis, Brown was awarded a $10,000 research grant (very large in those days) from NIH. In addition, the Eugene Meyer Foundation and the Veterans Administration supplemented the grant, making it possible to add the author, Dr. Harold Clark, a biochemist, to the research staff.

The rheumatoid arthritis patient's dream is to wake up some morning to a bright new day, pain free and rested. Several bright lights shining on the horizon may illuminate both the cause and the cure. Reports on the successful clinical trials of tetracycline (minocycline) in rheumatoid arthritis patients coming from several rheumatology clinics in the United Statets and other countries should definitely encourage other doctors to give it a try. The MIRA clinical trial concluded that "Patients who suffer from mild to moderate rheumatoid arthritis now have the choice of another therapeutic agent . . . . Not only did the antibiotic significantly reduce symptoms, but side effects were minimal and less severe than observed for most other common rheumatoid treatments" (Ann. Intern. Med., January, 1995).

With continued push and support from Congress, even more effective therapeutic modalities and antibiotics will be developed. Rheumatoid arthritis is a highly variable and individualized disorder representing only one branch of the highly complex rheumatic diseases. As most patients are hypersensitive, both the dosage and the drugs will have to be individually adjusted for each patient to achieve maximum benefits. The pharmaceutical companies, if there is enough profit, will be able to tailor safe new antibiotics directed toward both the infectious and symptomatic mechanisms as they have done for NSAIDS. Even today, many doctors still view tetracyclines strictly as antibiotics or antibacterial agents to be administered only after bacterial identification and in sufficient concentration to sustain effective blood levels and still avoid adverse side effects. Tetracyclines are now also recognized as chelating agents, which have several mechanisms of action, including anti-inflammatory, antioxidant, antimetabolic, immunosuppressive, and particularly their anticollagenase and antilysozomal enzyme activities. All of this adds up to a very broad spectrum antirheumatic drug, especially when administered as a multi-action drug. The ability of tetracyclines, alone or in combination with other anti-inflammatory drugs such as aspirin or ascorbic acid, to control (stop, reverse, prevent) rheumatoid disorders provides the all in one action. Unlike tetracyclines, the inability of other anti-inflammatory chelating agents, such as aspirin and ascorbic acid, to stop and maintain control of rheumatoid arthritis indicates their missing control of the persistent infectious cause. Whether persistent myoplasmas are the targeted causative agent in rheumatoid arthritis and other related disorders should soon be revealed.

The road is now open to the development and testing of even more effective antibiotics such as the erythromycin-like FK 506 drug, which also has very potent immunosuppressant activity and is made by a pharmaceutical company in Japan. This macrolide type antibiotic is being used primarily to block rejection in organ and tissue transplantation but is also being tested for use in certain autoimmune disorders, such as multiple sclerosis and diabetes. Hopefully, if its long-term side effects are not too great, it may prove to be another miracle drug against rheumatoid arthritis, Lupus, and other autoimmune diseases, including diabetes, multiple sclerosis, and Alzheimer's, whose infectious cause and cure are still unknown. Investigators soon may start testing the effectiveness of FK 506 in the spontaneous animal models, which will open the doors to the related human immunologic disorders. Perhaps investigators will now expand their search to include a possible role for mycoplasmas in these diseases, especially diabetes, which is also benefitted by tetracycline and FK 506 therapy. These common properties further suggest that other disorders could have similar disease mechanisms and causative agents.

Many chronic degenerative diseases, such as rheumatoid arthritis, are suspected of resulting from autoimmune or immune complex mechanisms of unknown infectious composition. The autoimmune disorders are comparable to the so-called Graft versus host reactions, where the host's immune system reacts against its own specific tissue components as though they were a foreign substance. The immune complex disorders are the inflammatory reactions that result when a foreign agent, such as a mycoplasma, is complexed with its antibody and becomes attached to specific host tissues, acting like an irritating thorn. Therefore, as previously found, neither the viable microbial agent nor its free antibodies would be readily associated with disease activity as long as they are kept separated by immunosuppressant drugs.

Mycoplasmas have frequently been associated with tissue autoanti-antibodies and tissue mimicry as well as immune complex disorders such as rheumatoid arthritis and Lupus. Mycoplasmas' persistent colonization (infectivity), which is clinically silent (asymptomatic) and common especially among females, has made their etiopathogenic (causative) mechanisms difficult to assess. The fact that mycoplasmas have frequently been associated with autoimmune activity and are known to elicit autoimmune reactions in animal models should definitely make them the first direction of future investigations.

Finding the great apes (gorilla, orangutan, chimpanzee) to be infected with and serologically expressing the human strains of mycoplasmas, as well as the anti-globulin rheumatoid factor, provides the ideal model of immunologically related rheumatoid disorders. The etiopathologic role of immune complexes in experimental vasculitis, especially the collagen vascular diseases, such as Lupus, with specific deposition on receptive kidney tissues, suggests that mycoplasmas could play a key role in other collagen vascular disorders. Our laboratory's identification of mycoplasma antigens in the immune complex fraction from rheumatoid arthritis patients' blood and joint fluid supports their role in immune complex disorders. As an immune complex, mycoplasmas attached to their antibodies, are neutralized (growth inhibited) but still remain viable and can activate the immune system, making them more difficult to isolate and detect. As antigen carriers, viable mycoplasmas bind and thus alter the attached host components, such as gamma globulin and myelin, making them autoantigens that are still able to be isolated.

Mycoplasmas have a high affinity and specificity for joint tissues and the vascular mucoproteins. Their specific binding and alteration of the attached basic proteins to form autoantigens provides them with a unique role as a persistent inflammatory autoimmune carrier. For example, by combining with and thus altering a host's mucoprotein, the host would form autoantibodies against its own vascular tissue mucoprotein. By combining with a basic myelin protein, mycoplasmas could thus induce autoantibodies against the myelin nerve sheath as in multiple sclerosis. By combining with a specific basic protein in the pancreatic beta cells, mycoplasmas could induce autoantibodies that would inhibit the insulin-producing cells as in diabetes.

This complexing and tissue binding provides an explanation for the inability to readily isolate mycoplasmas after initiating the immune disease mechanisms as well as their ubiquitous isolation from the nonreactive asymptomatic subjects. The genetic susceptibility factor plays a key role, as in other infectious processes, in determining who and what tissues become attached and the resulting disease. Like many of the autoimmune disorders, such as Alzheimer's, diabetes, multiple slcerosis, rheumatoid arthritis, and SLE, the slow erosion of specific functional tissues may occur over several years in the apparent absence of any detectable infectious agent and prior to any meaningful clinical expression. Thus the isolation frequency of mycoplasmas is not a sufficient criterion for establishing their pathogenic etiology. Researchers should realize that the older bacterial and viral concepts of infectious disease mechanisms do not apply to mycoplasmas. Immunologic disorders such as rheumatoid arthritis are the apparent symptoms resulting from the host's response to the irritant and not the resulting tissue destruction, as caused by bacterial or viral infections. Future investigations should now shift focus to the potential role of mycoplasmas as autoantigens and immune complexes in the chronic vascular pathogenesis of rheumatoid and other related disorders. In other words, mycoplasmas are not your typical infectious agent. These chronic disorders may not get the attention and support that the so-called killer diseases (heart, cancer, stroke, AIDS) receive but can inflict more damage and far greater cost, resulting in shorter life spans. How much brighter the future now looks for the millions who have waited patiently for the control and ultimate prevention of their disease.

It is truly unfortunate that the doctor who for over 40 years steadfastly pioneered and developed the antibiotic approach to the control of rheumatoid arthritis did not live to see his efforts fully materialize and be accepted. Why it took NIH and the American Rheumatism Association 40 years (1949-1989) to acknowledge and test Brown's hypothesis can never be justified when you consider the millions of patients who have suffered needlessly during this period. Perhaps a leading rheumatologist explained the reason best when he exclaimed "What are you guys trying to do—put us out of business?" I can only wonder how much longer they are going to drag their feet in testing and accepting a safer and more effective therapy for the countless millions of arthritics when the failure has been costing them untold billions for ineffective, stopgap, bandaid therapy. This medical disconcern makes you wonder how many other chronic disorders (heart, cancer, diabetes, multiple sclerosis) are being stonewalled for fear of clinics, institutes and foundations going out of business. The highly profitable pharmaceutical and insurance companies would have slim pickings if a cure was found for these diseases. Of course they will strongly oppose any health care program that will reduce the number of customers or the severity of medical problems.

Future Costs of Medical Research

What would you think if a director at NIH told you that NIH was chartered by Congress to conduct research and not to find the causes and cures of diseases? Perhaps it is time for Congress and the patients to find out who is responsible for finding the causes of their diseases as several billions of dollars are spent each year to develop more expensive diagnostic tests and palliative high-tech bandaid therapy. The cost of randomly searching for the cause and the cure is rapidly going out of reach.

Today's biotechnology in health and medicine has become profit motivated rather than problem solving. Consequently, the killer and crippling diseases—heart, cancer, arthritis, multiple sclerosis, diabetes, AIDS—remain rampant. Neither the Federal Government nor industry care to make the long-term costly investment that is necessary to find their primary causes rather than the more expensive stopgap therapy. With billions of dollars being spent each year for health and research and development, the solution and prevention of any one of our major diseases would yield far greater savings in our nation's and the world's economy.

One of the major problems many universities and medical schools now face is their becoming financially dependent on the industries and their applied research programs for greater support. Consequently, free and independent research has taken a backseat to patents and profits. Biotechnology such as genetic engineering has created new jobs and profits, but what about our nation's health? Has any major disease been eradicated recently?

Today we have reached the ridiculous pinnacle of medical research where the cure for a major disease has been found but is no longer profitable for distribution. In other words, the health industry's suppliers and providers will not be able to make as much profit as they do with the current ineffective and more toxic therapies. Consequently, the less profitable therapy, even though more beneficial, will not be tested or marketed.

Another example of today's health care crisis is the reduction and elimination of hospitalization motivated by the fallacious belief that it will reduce costs, regardless of solving chronic disease problems. Most doctors know from experience that there is no greater medicine than rest and relaxation free of stress. The most expensive medications and surgery cannot heal. Only the body can heal itself. Sending rheumatoid patients home to recover and heal would be exposing them to the same environment and conditions that could have initiated or precipitated the disorder. If it takes 10 times longer to recuperate at home, there certainly is no economic advantage. Our future health care program should consider rest as one of the most effective (and proven) forms of medication, especially for those chronic disease patients characterized by fatigue, anaemia, and lack of energy, which cannot be equated with cost or profit.

As a blue-ribbon arthritis committee pointed out over 20 years ago, that still holds true, "Today's therapy represents the sort of 'half-way' therapy medicine is obliged to adopt, as stopgap measures when the underlying mechanisms of the disease are still unknown. It is unlikely that we will be able to develop a genuinely effective treatment either for prevention or cure of the disease until these underlying mechanisms are clearly understood." The committee's first recommendation in 1972 was the "Identification of a possible viral-like agent as the cause of arthritis, as one of the most important lines of further study in arthritis research." Also in 1972, NIH was telling Congress that mycoplasmas should be investigated as a possible cause of rheumatoid arthritis. Patients should ask why over 99.5 percent of the NIH support is going in other directions.

Although it would be nearly impossible to identify and reassemble the many contributing links or reactants in the rheumatoid process, the elimination or breaking of a key link, such as the infectious agent (mycoplasmas), should effectively control and stop the disease mechanism. Stopping the symptoms does not stop the disease. Thus the theory behind the antimycoplasma therapeutic approach is to safely and effectively eliminate the infectious mycoplasmas as a most probable key link persisting in the reaction chain.

As we rapidly approach the 21st century and look back over our shoulder, we see the revolutionary technological advances that have been made in medicine, while the many chronic life-threatening disorders still remain with no known cause or cure. Applying some of these newer biotechnologies, we can now see that some antibiotics, like cortisone, are multiple edge swords and much more than just antibacterial agents. Mycoplasmas and even their genetic

192

fingerprints can now be seen in the tissues of patients with AIDS and other unsuspected places. Perhaps it is time we took mycoplasmas seriously and also took a look at the Alzheimer's, diabetes, and multiple sclerosis patients and even another look at cancer patients.

Although the pathologic reaction of mycoplasmas in rheumatoid arthritis remains unknown or hypothetical, their demonstrated presence in the host should require some remedial antibiotic therapy. As most medications, especially the newer and more potent ones, can have adverse accumulative reactions, the so called side effects, the pharmacologic basis of therapy has had to change. The doctor must balance tolerable versus effective individualized dosages and even pulsing doses on an intermittent daily or weekly basis, which gives the host cells a chance to catch their breath. Thus the inhibition of protein synthesis by tetracyclines can be adjusted to the host's response when a virulent infectious bacteria is not the primary target. As an antimycoplasma therapy, intermittent tetracycline doses can chip away at the persistent mycoplasmas without overwhelming the host's defense mechanisms. Even the anti-inflammatory medications, such as aspirin or ascorbic acid, could be beneficial by cooling the inflamed tissues and thus provide greater access and effectiveness for antimycoplasma therapy.

Prevention: An Ounce Is Worth a Ton of Cure

A prominent rheumatologist and tennis buff once told me that taking two aspirins before tackling strenuous exercises can prevent the resulting stiffness. This advice may remind you of the more famous study reporting that aspirin prevents heart disease. Also low cholesterol, low fat, and low salt diets and exercise have been strongly promoted to prevent cardiovascular disorders. Actually, these dietary and environmental changes more accurately reduce the incidence of the disease rather than preventing or eliminating its occurrence. If doctors are to prevent and eliminate the many unsolved chronic diseases (rheumatoid arthritis, SLE, multiple sclerosis, diabetes, Alzheimer's), therapy must be directed toward eradicating the early primary cause and not just the resulting symptoms and numerous contributing factors. The research team of biochemists, immunologists, microbiologists, physicians, and others, must review and take a fresh look at the very broad gap between the onset and the clinical diagnosis of a disease or syndrome. What is early rheumatoid arthritis? When the patients first feel an ache or fatigue? The team must first determine how and why that first infectious agent (such as mycoplasma) attaches to or enters the first tissue cell without expressing any clinical symptoms. In addition to different genetic types and thousands of other predisposing and contributing factors, the infectious agent and host cell begin their fight for survival. The course and severity of the fight depends on which cells and what tissues are infected (blood cells or synovial tissue cells) and the particular type of infectious agent. As the fight proliferates and more cells and more microbes are involved, the microscopic analysis of the tissue section may eventually reveal cellular changes. These changes may take the form of minimal cellular aggregation or destruction depending upon how active and irritating the infectious agent is.

If the fight ends there, it is considered subclinical with no medication prescribed. If the fight reoccurs or persists with greater cellular activity and destruction, producing pain and swelling (symptoms), it is considered a clinical expression and requires aspirin or antibiotic therapy for relief and control. The only problem is that once the fight or disease reaches the surface, it may become a self-sustaining cellular battle with antibiotic therapy having less effect on reaching the mycoplasma or infectious agent or stopping the disease. As demonstrated in both animal models and humans, once the mycoplasma-cellular fight reaches the surface to produce arthritis or pneumonia, the antibiotic (tetracycline) therapy is less effective on the course of the disease.

Insulin-dependent diabetes is another good example of a delayed subclinical disease onset, where the infectious agent and autoimmune response may take several years before the insulin-producing pancreatic Beta cells are sufficiently damaged to cause the insulin deficiency symptomatic diabetes response with extensive peripheral vascular destruction.

Based on present-day evidence and not knowing when first exposed to the infectious cause, such as mycoplasmas, it would seem prudent and advisable for doctors to routinely test for mycoplasma antibodies as they do for Lyme disease. A positive test would indicate a fight has begun, even if it has not surfaced, and thus indicate

194

the need for early and effective antimycoplasma therapy. Finding a cure and early prevention for rheumatic diseases will make the future much brighter for millions. Now being able to utilize an ounce of preventive therapy should make it possible to provide an arthritis-free future.

The green light is on, the doors are open, and the solution and answers to arthritis are now in the hands of the doctors. Fortunately, some doctors are already headed in the antibiotic direction and are now providing many rheumatoid patients with a brighter and pain-free future, while many more doctors may follow.

Update: The Beginning of the End to Arthritis.
Both patients and doctors will now be looking at the results of the minocycline trial by the six clinical centers that was supported by NIH and published in the Annals of Internal Medicine in January, 1995. The report concluded that "Patients who suffer from mild to moderate rheumatoid arthritis now have the choice of another effective and safe therapeutic agent [minocycline]." The investigators further concluded that "Not only did the antibiotic significantly reduce symptoms, but side effects were minimal and less severe than observed for most other common rheumatoid arthritis treatments."

Apparently the Arthritis Foundation was still not impressed with the demonstration of a safer and effective alternative therapy. The foundation's medical director said that he would not call it a breakthrough and that more study of dosages and long-term use of minocycline is needed.

One doctor who had previously reported that tetracycline treatment was not effective in rheumatoid arthritis now indicated that "It may be that Dr. Brown was giving the drug (tetracycline) for the wrong reasons and in the wrong doses", instead of admitting that he had wronged the arthritis patients—and not Dr. Brown.

In reporting their findings to the news media, the clinical investigators erroneously told the public that the minocycline study is the first use of antibiotics against rheumatoid arthritis. They must know that this was a false and misleading statement as antibiotics, especially the tetracyclines, have been used to treat rheumatoid arthritis since they were first introduced in 1947. The Lederle

195

Co., which provided the minocycline for their clinical trial, also provided Brown with Aureomycinin 1947 to treat rheumatoid patients. The results of this first trial of tetracycline in 17 patients were reported by Brown in 1949 at the National Arthritis meeting in New York City, the same meeting where the beneficial effects of cortisone were being introduced. Two years later (1951) Brown and his associates published further beneficial results on the effectiveness of three other antibiotics in the *American Journal of Medical Sciences*. This report also included the administration of intravenous antibiotics that they believed were targeting virus-like organisms (mycoplasmas) known to cause arthritis in animals.

Supported by a grant from NIH, Duke University Medical Center is now testing the effectiveness of intravenous tetracycline therapy in rheumatoid arthritis, which was first proposed and successfully used by Brown. Now using costly and ultra-sensitive techniques, an all-out effort has been launched by NIH to find the infective causes of rheumatoid arthritis by examining synovial tissues at the earliest stage possible. Although it will be a most difficult and complex task, hopefully the investigators will succeed in finding the prevention for rheumatoid arthritis and related disorders. Thus we will have answers to Why Arthritis?

196

About the Author

Harold W. Clark, Ph. D., has spent more than 40 years investigating the probable causes and cures of rheumatoid diseases. His primary theme has been the role and mechanism of mycoplasmas in rheumatoid diseases, including those in humans, gorillas, and elephants, often introducing and defending new evidence to support the cause and cure. He has taken his scientific message to such countries as Scotland, Finland, France, Germany, Sweden, Egypt, Brazil, the Philippines, Australia, Thailand, Japan, and Mexico. Scientific publications from his years of research have been disseminated and translated worldwide, and now his book, *Why Arthritis?*, explores and documents 40-year development of the safe and effective antibiotic treatment and probable infectious cause. The author has held positions as both Associate Research Professor of Medicine, and as Research Director of the Medical Rehabilitation Center at George Washington University, Washington, D.C., and was Research Director and Vice-Chairman of the Arthritis Institute of the National Hospital, Arlington, VA. He is presently Director of the Mycoplasma Research Institute. His current memberships include the International Organization for Mycoplasmologists, the American Society for Microbiology, and the American Association for the Advancement of Science.

THE ARTHRITIS INSTITUTE'S ROLE IN THE SEARCH FOR THE CAUSE AND CURE OF RHEUMATOID ARTHRITIS

1939   First to report the isolation of Mycoplasmas (PPLO) from rheumatic tissues and fluids. Science 89:271-272, 1939. Brown, et.al.

1949   First to report on the successful use of tetracycline in the treatment of Rheumatic Diseases. J. Lab. Clin. Med. 34:1404-1410, 1949. Brown, et.al.

1951   First to report on the successful use of intravenous tetracycline in the treatment of Rheumatic Diseases. Amer. J. Med. Sci. 221:618-625, 1951. Brown, et.al.

1956   First to report the Contamination of Human Cell Cultures by Mycoplasmas (PPLO). Science 124:(3232), 1147-1148, 1956. Robinson, et.al.

1965   First to report finding Mycoplasma antibodies in rheumatoid arthritis patients. Fifth Interscience Conference, Washington D.C. 1965. Clark, et.al.

1966   First to report the localization of Mycoplasma antibodies in the joint fluids from rheumatoid arthritis patients. Arthritis & Rheumatism 9:495, 1966. Clark, et.al.

1969   First to isolate Mycoplasma from and successfully treat a rheumatoid gorilla with I.V. tetracycline. Trans. Amer. Clin. & Climatol. Assoc. 82:227-247, 1969. Brown, et.al.

1978   First to isolate new Mycoplasma species from rheumatoid elephants and treat them with antibiotic therapy. J. Zoo Anim. Med. 11:3-15, 1980. Clark, et.al.

1982   First to show 5 year sustained improvement in rheumatoid patients and gorilla models using an antibiotic approach to treatment. in "Inflammatory Diseases & Copper", Ed. JRJ Sorenson, Humana press, 391-407, 1982. Brown, et.al.

1988   First to report finding Mycoplasma antigens in the Immune Complex from rheumatoid joint fluid and sera. Annals of Allergy, 60:394-398, 1988. Clark, et.al.

1991   First to identify a Mycoplasma cause of the anti-IgG rheumatoid-like factor. Amer. J. Primatology, 24:235-243, 1991. Clark, et.al.

APPENDIX

Correspondence

THE WHITE HOUSE

WASHINGTON

April 6, 1977

Dear Dr. Clark:

The President has asked me to thank you for your kind invitation to attend the IXVth International Congress of Rheumatology to be held in San Francisco on June 26.

As much as he appreciates your thoughtfulness in offering him this opportunity and would like to be able to join you, the President has such a heavy schedule outlined that he will be unable to add this engagement to his commitments. He does want you to know, though, of his warm appreciation to you for inviting him and that he sends his very best wishes to you, particularly for a most successful conference.

Sincerely,

Fran Voorde
Director of Scheduling

Harold W. Clark, Ph.D.
Director of Research
The Arthritis Institute
    of the National Orthopaedic
    Rehabilitation Hospital
2455 Army Navy Drive
Arlington, Virginia 22206

Correspondence

November 21, 1969

Dear Dr. Clark:

The President forwarded your letter of November 14 to me. Since I was involved in Dr. Brown's visit with the late President Eisenhower, I was more than casually interested in your letter and the report you enclosed. Dr. Brown is to be congratulated for the fine work that he has done in arthritis research.

The President wishes to thank you and to extend his best wishes for continued success in the treatment of arthritis.

Sincerely,

Walter R. Tkach
Colonel, USAF, MC
Physician to the President

Harold W. Clark, Ph.D.
Associate Research Professor of Medicine (Biochemistry)
The George Washington University Medical Center
2150 Pennsylvania Avenue, N.W.
Washington, D.C. 20037

Correspondence

HARVARD MEDICAL SCHOOL

RUTH B. KUNDSIN, Sc.D.
*Associate Professor of Microbiology
and Molecular Genetics*

BRIGHAM AND WOMEN'S HOSPITAL

75 Francis Street
Boston, Massachusetts 02115
617-732-6410

Sept 4, 1991

Dear Harold,

Was I ever glad to hear from you — and I think your paper is terrific. I have copied it and sent it to several colleagues. I have a paper with Peter Schur an authority on SLE and RA — I sent him a copy and also to a young Ethiopian doctor who is brilliant and has been interested in the impact of mycoplasmas on T cells. You should come to meeting. I'd like to see you. Do you ever get up to Boston? I'm also referencing your paper in a grant proposal which I don't imagine I'll get — but it's fun putting it together. I loved your statement that my coplasmas

Correspondence

Are "undercover agents" — I'm going to
use that in the grant proposal —
indicating they are very insidious.
I'm extremely pleased that you are
continuing your my explained work.
Write & tell me what you are doing.

All best and thanks
for the reprint —
Ruth

P.S. Are you OK? I am —

Correspondence

CORNELL UNIVERSITY MEDICAL COLLEGE
1300 YORK AVENUE NEW YORK, N.Y. 10021
(212) 746-6595

SCHOLAR-IN-RESIDENCE
ROOM #734

May 16, 1989

Dr. Harold W. Clark
Mycoplasma Research Institute
2117 Reynolds Street
Falls Church, VA 22043

Dear Dr. Clark:

Thank you for your April 25 letter, and my apologies
for the delay. I was extremely sorry to learn of Tom
Brown's death. I had known him since my brief years at
Hopkins just after the war, and followed his published
work with keen interest. I'm glad to see that the
mycoplasma continues to be under puzzled scrutiny in
various laboratories, and I continue to have high hopes
for its future (although in recent years I've also laid
a few small bets on L-forms).

Warm regards.

Yours,

Lewis Thomas

Lewis Thomas, M.D.

LT/sh

206

T. L. SCHULTE, A.B., (ZOOLOGY) M.D., M.S., (UROLOGY)
219 FAMILY FARM DRIVE, WOODSIDE, CALIFORNIA 94062
PHONE 415-851-0520   FAX 415-851-8278

Sept 20, 1991

Dear Harold,

Thank you for your excellent paper "The potential role of Mycoplasmas as Autoantigens and immune Complexes in Chronic Vascular Pathogenesis".

I have been working with superoxide dismutase for the past 30 years and find that it seems to be an indirect measure of allergies, antiinflammatory and immune measurement. The use of SOD also prevents scar tissue formation even as long as after 40 yrs. SOD seems to effect the collagen metabolism thus preventing scar tissue formation.

I am attempting to measure free radicals, specifically superoxide, in the serum or plasma, in order to get a comparable measure for comparison of source material compared to physiological effectiveness. Perhaps somewhere along the line Mycoplasmas may be a factor.

Thank you again for your reprint.

Most sincerely,

Tom

Correspondence

The Warren Grant Magnuson Clinical Center

Department of Health
and Human Services

Building 10, Room 2C146
National Institutes of Health
Bethesda, Maryland 20892
Telephone 301-496-4114

October 17, 1989

Harold W. Clark, PhD
2117 Reynolds Street
Falls Church, VA 22043

Dear Harold:

Thank you for your note of October 10th and the interesting abstract from the Rio meeting.

As you probably know, I am now Director of the Clinical Center and have not fooled around in arthritis research let alone mycoplasma work for 6 years now. Nonetheless, as you can imagine, arthritoid ideas are still of great interest to me.

I would certainly appreciate receiving a copy (either as a preprint or reprint) of the publication, "The Potential Role of Mycoplasmas as Autoantigens and Immune Complexes in Chronic Vascular Pathogenesis."

Cordially yours,

John L. Decker, M.D.
Director, Clinical Center

Correspondence

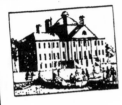

MASSACHUSETTS GENERAL HOSPITAL

J. ROBERT BUCHANAN, M.D.
General Director

Boston. 02114
Telephone (617) 726-_____

Cable Address "Massgenral"

Dr. Harold W Clark

Dear Harold:

I am so glad to hear that you are still working with Mycoplasma at the Research Institute. Is this a new Center or has it been going on for a long while? Your work is fascinating and opens up new potentialities for the role of mycoplasmas in   auto immune disorders. Unfortunately I am not sophisticated enough in this area to pursue such studies, but I am always anxious to know everything that is done with them and about them, as you know. If you are ever up in the Boston area again, you must come and talk to the L.D. Study Group again.

With kindest personal regards and keep up the good work.

Sincerely yours,

Sarabelle Madoff

Correspondence

DEPARTMENT OF HEALTH & HUMAN SERVICES

Public Health Service
National Institutes of Health

National Institute of Arthritis and
Musculoskeletal and Skin Diseases
Bethesda, Maryland 20892
Building: 31
Room: 9A-35
(301) 496-

September 20, 1988

Dr. Harold W. Clark
Mycoplasma Research Institute
2117 Reynolds Street
Falls Church, VA 22043

Dear Harold:

Thanks so much for your very good letter of September 14. I am very pleased to know about your current activities and that you will be available as a consultant in the important area of mycoplasma and immunological and arthritis research.

Thank you very much for enclosing your interesting reprint from the "Annals of Allergy" this past May.

I will be pleased to place your name on our Institute's mailing list.

With all best wishes to you.

Sincerely,

Lawrence E. Shulman, M.D., Ph.D.
Director
National Institute of Arthritis and
Musculoskeletal and Skin Diseases

cc: Ms. Constance D. Raab

Correspondence

The University of Alabama at Birmingham
School of Medicine/Department of Medicine
J. Claude Bennett, M.D.
Professor and Chairman
Physician-in-Chief
University of Alabama Hospital
205/934-7400
FAX 205/934-1477
Telex: 888826 UAB BHM

November 13, 1989

Harold W. Clark, Ph.D.
Mycoplasma Research Institute
2117 Reynolds St.
Falls Church, VA 22043

Dear Dr. Clark:

Thank you very much for your note of October 27 and a copy of your abstract "Mycoplasma Bound IgG Expresses Autoantigenic anti-idiotypic antibodies".

Of course, I am very much interested in your work and would appreciate reprints or preprints of any publications which you have in press on this exciting area.

With best regards,

sincerely yours,

J. Claude Bennett

J. Claude Bennett, M.D.

JCB:eb

Correspondence

NationalCancerAdvisoryBoard

National Cancer Institute

Bethesda, Maryland 20205

National Cancer Program

Reply To:
Hon. Tim Lee Carter M.D.
Tompkinsville, Ky. 42167
(502) 487-8696 or (202) 332-7700

July 29, 1983

Thomas McPherson Brown, M.D.
Chairman
The Arthritis Institute
2455 Army Navy Drive
Arlington, Virginia 22206

Dear Dr. Brown:

I want you to know I appreciate your excellent work, and by using your methods it has been possible for me to obtain a remission for a 12 year old youngster. He later served in our airforce for 2½ years.

Your work to me shows more promise then any other researcher or physician in the field of arthritis.

You have also appeared before committees in Congress on which I served on more than one occasion. I have tremendous respect and admiration for your work.

Sincerely yours,

National Cancer Advisory Board

Tim Lee Carter, M.D.
Chairman

Correspondence

THE SECRETARY OF THE INTERIOR
WASHINGTON

March 23, 1984

Dr. Thomas McP. Brown
The Arthritis Clinic
   of Northern Virginia
2465 Army-Navy Drive
Arlington, Virginia 22206

Dear Tom:

Thank you so much for your letter of the 14th, which Joan and I have studied carefully.

In far greater gratitude, I thank you for the foresight, research and counsel that led me to recover from an affliction that literally had me on my back a few years ago. I shall continue in my support in every way I can of your great work.

Sincerely,

William Clark

Correspondence

THE SECRETARY OF HEALTH AND HUMAN SERVICES
WASHINGTON, D.C. 20201

April 6, 1983

Harold W. Clark, Ph.D.
Director of Research
The Arthritis Institute
of the National Hospital
2455 Army Navy Drive
Arlington, Virginia 22206

Dear Dr. Clark:

Thank you for your thoughtful and informative letter. Your words of support are indeed encouraging.

As you know, my deep commitment and sympathy towards sufferers of arthritis are longstanding. I regard this debilitating disease as a major health challenge and a top priority to which this Department will address itself.

I look forward to working with you.

Sincerely,

Margaret Heckler

Margaret M. Heckler
Secretary

214

Correspondence

TAMPEREEN YLIOPISTO
BIOLÄÄKETIETEEN LAITOS

UNIVERSITY OF TAMPERE
DEPARTMENT OF BIOMEDICAL SCIENC

February 13, 1992

Dr. Harold W. Clark
Mycoplasma Research Institute
P.O. Box 40
Beverly Hills
FLORIDA 32665-0040

Dear Harold:

Happy New Year 1992 to you and Bonnie.

Thank you very much for your interesting letter which arrived already in January. At that time I was very busy teaching medical students, for the last time. I am namely retiring at the end of this year.

Hopefully many other doctors will continue where Dr. Brown and you have left.

With best wishes to you and Bonnie,

Yours sincerely,

Elli Jansson, M.D.

POSTIOSOITE:
PL 607
33101 TAMPERE

TAY 0.091a

KATUOSOITE:
Laäkärinkatu 3
Tampere

PUH/TEL: (931) 156 111
TELEX 22415 layki sf
TELEFAX +358 31 156 170

BOX 607
SF-33101 TAMPERE
FINLAND

215

Correspondence

MINISTRY OF CULTURE
ANTIQUTIES ORGANIZATION
EGYPTIAN MUSEUM

28 / 8 / 1995

Harold W. Clark
MACOPLASMA RESEARCH INSTITUTE

Dear Director, Clark

In reply to your letter to H.E. the Cultural and Educational councelar of the Embassy of the A.R.E in Washington, D.C. dated in August 8 , 1995. We would like to inform you that permission is granted to publish the photograph of the servant brewing from our museum in the book .

Best Wishes

Dr. Mohamed Saleh

Director

The Egyptian Museum

216

Correspondence

Embassy of The Arab Republic of Egypt
Cultural and Educational Bureau

September 15, 1995

Dr. Harold W. Clark
Director
Mycoplasma Research Institute
P.O. Box 640040
Beverly Hills, Florida 34464-0040

Dear Dr. Clark:

I am writing this letter regarding your request to the Egyptian Museum to use a copy of an artwork which is located in the museum. Your request was sent to Egypt by this office and I am happy to inform you that permission has been granted.

The letter from the museum giving you authorization to use the photograph is attached. I wish you much success in your endeavor to find a cure for arthritis.

Sincerely yours,

Dr. Abdul-Monem Al-Mashat
Director

1303 New Hampshire Ave., N.W. Washington, D.C. 20036
Tel: (202) 296-3888 • Fax: (202) 296-3891 • E-Mail: 54887480.MCI.Mail.Com

American College of Rheumatology

NEWS RELEASE

Media Notice

Two studies on the effect of the antibiotic minocycline on rheumatoid arthritis will be presented at the American College of Rheumatology Annual Scientific Meeting Nov. 8 in San Antonio, Texas

The authors of these papers will brief the media at 1:30 CST at the San Antonio Convention Center.

An expert on this subject will be available to comment on these studies after the briefing. To set up an interview, call the press room at (210) 270-2923 Nov. 7-11.

Background

In 1988, researcher Thomas McPherson Brown, MD, published *The Road Back*, a book documenting that minocycline was effective in the treatment of rheumatoid arthritis. Most researchers felt that the methods used to conduct the study were not adequate to support the claims. Dr. Brown died before he could conduct further research.

Since then, the National Institute for Arthritis and Musculoskeletal and Skin Diseases, a branch of the National Institutes of Health, funded a study on minocycline. A group of Dutch researchers also investigated the effect of minocycline on rheumatoid arthritis.

The Dutch study concludes that minocycline is safe and beneficial in the treatment of rheumatoid arthritis. Considerable improvement was seen in 43 percent of the people taking minocycline while none showed considerable deterioration.

The results of the U.S. study will be presented Nov. 8 in San Antonio.

Transcription of Speech by:
Caspar Weinberger
Secretary of Defense

Secretary Weinberger: It is a great privilege to have the opportunity to share with all of you in the much deserved tributes to Dr. Brown. Ordinarily I don't read my speeches but this is a special exception as this isn't one of my speeches. This is a message from the President and I am delighted to have the opportunity to read it:

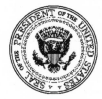

October 16, 1982

"Dear Doctor Brown:

I am pleased to extend congratulations to you as you reach your 50th year of medical service. Your accomplishments, both as a practicing physician and as an authority on arthritis, are widely known and valued, and your leadership in clinical practice and research has been responsible for reducing the suffering of arthritis victims throughout the world. Your contributions to making this nation a healthier place to live are greatly appreciated. I wish you many more years of happiness in your endeavors."

Sincerely,

Ronald Reagan
President of the United States

REFERENCES

American Rheumatism Association: Dear Colleague; Rheumatoid Arthritis— Causes and Treatment, Letter, April 14, 1988

Anastassiades TP: Remission-inducing drugs in rheumatoid arthritis. Can Med Assoc J 122: 405-415, 1980

Arthritis Foundation: Basic Facts. New York, NY, The Arthritis Foundation 1976 U.S. Congress: The National Arthritis Act, P.L. 93-640, January 4, 1975

Arthritis Foundation: Promising therapies of the 90's: Arthritis research enters a new decade. Arthritis Today, February 1990

Arthritis, Rheumatic Diseases, and Related Disorders, 1993 Research Highlights. NIH Publication No. 93-3413, 1993

Bassett EJ, Keith MS, Armelagos GJ, Martin DL, Villanueva AR: Tetracycline-labeled human bone from ancient Sudanese Nubia (A.D.350). Science 209:1532-1534, 1980

Breedveld FC, Dijkmans BA, Mattie H: Minocycline treatment for rheumatoid arthritis; An open dose finding study. J Rheumatol 17:43-46, 1990

Brown TMcP, Bailey JS, Iden KI, Clark HW: Antimycoplasma approach to the mechanism and the control of rheumatoid disease. In: Inflammatory Diseases and Copper, JRJ Sorenson, ed. Clifton, New Jersey, Humana Press, 1982, 391-407

Brown TMcP, Clark HW, Bailey JS: Rheumatoid arthritis in the gorilla: A study of Mycoplasma-host interaction in pathogenesis and treatment. In: Comparative Pathology of Zoo Animals, eds. Montali RJ, Magaki G. Wash. DC, Smithsonian Institution Press, 1980, 259-266

Brown TMcP, Clark HW, Bailey JS: The isolation of mycoplasma from pleural fluid in rheumatoid arthritis. 13th International Congress of Rheumatology, Japan, 1973. Excerpta Medica, Abstract 594

Brown TMcP: Discussion. In: Rheumatic Diseases, Seventh International Congress on Rheumatic Disease. Philadelphia, WB Saunders, 1952, 407-408

Brown TMcP, Scammell H: The Road Back—Rheumatoid Arthritis—Its Cause and Its Treatment. New York, M. Evans & Co., 1988

Brown TMcP, Wichelhausen RH, Merchant WR, Robinson LB: A study of the antigen-antibody mechanism in rheumatic diseases. Am J Med Sci 221:618-625, 1951

Brown TMcP, Wichelhausen RH, Robinson LB, Merchant WR: The in vivo action of aureomycin on pleuropneumonia-like organisms associated with various rheumatic diseases. J Lab Clin Med 34: 1404-1414, 1949

Cassell GH, Cole BC: Future research directions—Mycoplasmas as agents of human disease. N Engl J Med 304:80-89,1981

Catterall A: Legg-Calve-Perthes' syndrome. Clin Orthop 158:41-52, 1981

Chanock RM, Hayflick L, Barile, MF: Growth on artificial medium of an agent associated with atypical pneumonia and its identification as a PPLO. Proc Natl Acad Sci USA 48:41-49, 1962

Clark HW, Bailey JS, Brown TMcP: Properties supporting the role of mycoplasmas in rheumatoid arthritis. Rev Infect Dis 4:S238-239, 1982

Clark HW, Brown TMcP: Another look at mycoplasmas. Arthritis Rheum 19:649-650,1976

Clark HW, Brown TMcP: The antimycoplasma approach to the treatment of rheumatoid arthritis. In: Part 9 Hearings before the House Appropriations subcommittee 1984, 714-741

Clark HW: Letter to editor. Ann Intern Med 123:393, 1995

Clark HW: The potential role of mycoplasmas as autoantigens and immune-complexes in chronic vascular pathogenesis. Am J Primatol 24:235-243, 1991

Cooperman Y: Avoiding quackery in arthritis. In: Aches and Pains. UK, Geigy Pharmaceuticals, June 1981

Cousins N: Anatomy of an Illness as Perceived by the Patient: Reflections on Healing and Regeneration. New York, Norton, 1979

Decker JL, Barden JA: *Mycoplasma hyorhinis* arthritis of swine: A model of rheumatoid arthritis. In: Immunological Aspects of Rheumatoid Arthritis. Rheumatology, Volume 6. Basel, Karger, 1975

Decker JL: Rheumatoid arthritis: Evolving concepts of pathogenesis and treatment. Ann Intern Med 101:810-824, 1984

Decker JL: The Relationship of Mycoplasma to Rheumatoid Arthritis and Related Diseases, Proceedings of the Conference. NIH Public Health Service Publication No. 1523, 1966

Dienes L, Edsall G: Observations on L organisms of Klieneberger. Proc Soc Exp Biol Med 36:740-744, 1937

Dienes L, Ropes MW, Smith WE, Madoff S, Bauer W: The role of pleuropneumonia-like organisms in genitourinary and joint diseases. N Engl J Med 238:509-515, 1948

Dienes L, Weinberger HJ: Experimental arthritis— Pleuropneumonia-like organisms and their possible relation to articular disease. In: Rheumatic Diseases, Seventh International Congress on Rheumatic Diseases. Philadelphia WB Saunders, 1952, 401-406

Findlay GM, Mackenzie RD, MacCallum FO, Klieneberger E: The etiology of polyarthritis in the rat. Lancet 2:7-10, 1939

Fuerst ML: The arthritis-infection connection: Skeptics reconsider. Medical World News September 9, 1985

Hakkarainen K, Turunen H, Miettinen A, Karppelin M, Kaitila K, Jansson E: Mycoplasmas and arthritis. Ann Rheum Dis 51:1170-1172, 1992

Hannan PC: Sodium aurothiomalate, gold keratinate, and various tetracyclines in mycoplasma-induced arthritis of rodents. J Med Microbiol 10:87-102,1977

Harris ED Jr: Mycoplasma and Arthritis, A Report to the National Arthritis Advisory Board, October 21, 1983

Hart FD: History of the treatment of rheumatoid arthritis. British Medical Journal, 27 March 1976

Jackson FL: Mode of action of tetracyclines. In: Experimental Chemotherapy, Vol. 3, Schnitzer RJ, Hawking F, ed. New York, Academic Press, 1964, 71-101

Kay JE, Senam E, Doe A, Benzie CR: The mechanism of action of the immunosuppressive drug FK-506. Cell Immunol 124:175-181, 1989

Kloppenburg M, Breedveld FC, Terwiel JP, Mallee C, Dijkmans BA: Minocycline in active rheumatoid arthritis. A double-blind, placebo-controlled trial. Arthritis Rheum 37:629-636, 1994

Kundsin RB, Driscoll SG, Praznik J: The role of mycoplasmas in spontaneous abortion. In: Mycoplasma Diseases of Man,

Proceedings of International Symposium, Rheinhardsbrunn Castle, Sprossig M, Witzleb W, eds. VEB Gustov Fischer Verlag, Jena, 1969, 141-148 German Democratic Republic

Langevitz P, Bank I, Zemer D, Book M, Pras M: Treatment of resistant rheumatoid arthritis with minocycline: An open study. J Rheumatol 19:1502-1504, 1992

Lockshin MD: The Unproven Remedies Committee. Arthritis Rheum 24:1188-1190, September 1981

National Commission on Arthritis and Related Musculoskeletal Diseases: Report to the Congress of the United States, Volume I. The Arthritis Plan. DHEW Publication No. (NIH) 76-1150, 1976 Bethesda, MD

National Institutes of Health: NIH Report: Mycoplasma Research, Infectious Disease Theory Research, or Antibiotic Clinical Trials, A Ten Year (1982-1992) Report in Response to Senate Report 102-397, January 1993

NIH Conference: The Role of Infectious Agents and Immunologic Reactions in the Genesis of Chronic and Degenerative Diseases of Man, October 1965, Bethesda, MD

NIH News Release: Susceptibility to arthritis linked to brain's regulation of inflammation. Pro Natl Acad Sci USA, April 1989

NIH Response Report No. 97-894: Mycoplasmas and antimycoplasmal treatment: A review of their role in rheumatoid arthritis. In: Part 9 Hearings Before House Appropriations Subcommittee 1984, 692-713

NIH Response to Senate Report No. 97-680: Report on Mycoplasmas, Antimycoplasma Therapy, and Rheumatoid Arthritis. December 1983

Nocard E, Roux ER, et al.: Le microbe de la peripeumonie. Ann Ins

224

Pasteur 12:240-262, 1898

Robinson LB, Wichelhausen RH, Roisman B: Contamination of human cell cultures by pleuropneumonia-like organisms. Science 124:1147-1149, 1956

Sabin AB: Identification of the filtrable transmissible neurolytic agent isolated from toxoplasma-infected tissue as a new pleuropneumonia-like microbe. Science 88:575-576, 1938

Schumacher HR Jr, Klippel JH, Koopman WJ: Primer on the Rheumatic Diseases, Tenth Edition. Atlanta, Arthritis Foundation, 1993

Sharp JT, Lidsky MD, Duffy J: Clinical responses during gold therapy for rheumatoid arthritis. Arthritis Rheum 25:540-549, 1982

Short CL, Dienes L, Bauer W: Autogenous vaccines in rheumatoid arthritis. Am J Med Sci 187:615-623, 1934

Skinner M, Cathcart ES, Mills JA, Pinals RS: Tetracycline in the treatment of rheumatoid arthritis. A double blind controlled study. Arthritis Rheum 14:727-732, 1971

Smith CB, Friedewald WT, Chanock RM: Shedding of mycoplasma pneumoniae after tetracycline and erythromycin therapy. N Engl J Med 276:1172-1175, 1966

Sorenson JRJ: Copper complexes offer a physiological approach to treatment of chronic diseases. In: Progress in Medicinal Chemistry, Vol 26, Ellis GP, West GB, eds. Elsevier Science Publishers, B.V. Amsterdam, 1989, 437-568

Sterner G, Biberfeld G: Central nervous complications of mycoplasma pneumoniae infection. Scand J Infect Dis 1:203-208, 1969

Swift HF, Brown TMcP: Pathogenic pleuropneumonia-like

organisms from rheumatic exudates and tissues. Science 89:271-272, 1939

Thomas L: New Directions in Arthritis Research. New York, Arthritis Foundation Report, 1973

Thomas L: The Youngest Science: Notes of a Medicine Watcher. New York, Viking Press, 1983

Tilley BC, Alarcon GS, Heyse S, Trentham DE, Neuner R, Kaplan DA, et al.: Minocycline in rheumatoid arthritis. A 48-week double-blind, placebo-controlled trial. Ann Intern Med 122:81-89, 1995

U.S. House of Representatives: Request for Report No. 97-894, H.R. 7205, 1983

U.S. Senate Report No.97-680: Request for NIH report on: Mycoplasmas, antimycoplasma therapy, and rheumatoid arthritis. In: FY 1983 Appropriations Bill. Congressional Record S14144, December 8, 1982

Walker WR: The results of a copper bracelet clinical trial and subsequent studies. In: Inflammatory Diseases and Copper, JRJ Sorenson, ed. Clifton, New Jersey, Humana Press, 1982, 469-482

Wolf B: Therapy of inflammatory Diseases with superoxide dismutase. In: Inflammatory Diseases and Copper, JRJ Sorenson, ed. Clifton, New Jersey, Humana Press, 1982, 453-467

World Health Organization: The Role of Immune Complexes in Disease. Technical Report Series 606, 1977

Publications By The Author

1. Clark HW, Dounce AL, Stotz E: An improved method for the extraction and purification of diphosphopyridine nucleotide. J. Biol. Chem. 181:459-466, 1949.
2. Clark HW: Succinic Dehydrogenase - Cytochrome-c link in heart muscle succinoxidase. Fed. Proc. 9:160, 1950.
3. Clark HW, Neufeld HA, Widmer C, Stotz E: Purification of a factor linking succinic dehydrogenase with cytochrome-c. J. Biol. Chem. 210:851-860, 1954.
4. Clark HW, Neufeld HA, Widmer C, Stotz E: Cytochrome-b. Fed. Proc. 10:172, 1951.
5. Widmer CH, Clark HW, Nufeld HA, Stotz E: Cytochrome components of the soluble SC factor preparation. J. Biol. Chem. 210:861-867, 1954.
6. Wichelhausen RH, Clark HW, Griffing VF, Robinson LB: The property of human serum albumin to conceal visible evidence of bacterial contamination. Am. J. Med. 20:957, 1956.
7. Wichelhausen RH, Clark HW, Griffing VF, Robinson LB: The concealment of heavy bacterial contamination in 25 percent human serum albunin. J. Lab. Clin. Med. 51:276-287, 1958.
8. Clark HW, Wichelhausen RH, Brown TMcP: Standardization of serum protein analysis by paper electrophoresis. Fed. Proc. 17:202, 1958.
9. Clark HW, Fowler RC, Brown TMcP: Preparation of pleuro-pneumonia-like organisms for microscopic study. J. Bacteriol. 81:500-502, 1961.
10. Bailey JS, Clark HW, Felts WR, Fowler RC, Brown TMcP: Antigenic properties of pleuropneumonia-like organisms from tissue cell cultures and the human genital area. J. Bacteriol. 82:542-547, 1961.
11. Clark HW: Figure of a mycoplasma colony in Fundamentals of Microbiology, 7th edition, Frobisher, M, ed. WB Saunders, 1962.
12. Clark HW, Bailey JS, Fowler RC, Brown TMcP: Identification

of mycoplasmatacea by the fluorescent antibody method. J. Bacteriol. 85:111-118, 1963.

13. Bailey JS, Clark HW, Felts WR, Brown TMcP: Growth inhibitory properties of mycoplasma antibody. J. Bacteriol. 86: 147-150, 1963.

14. Clark HW, Bailey JS, Brown TMcP: Determination of mycoplasma antibodies in humans. Bacteriol. Proc. 64:59 M87, 1964.

15. Clark, HW: Figure of a mycoplasma colony. In Zinsser Microbiology, 13th edition, Smith OT, Conant NF, Overman JR, ed. Appleton-Century-Crofts, Inc., 1964.

16. Clark HW: Sedimentation counting and morphology of mycoplasma. J. Bacteriol. 90: 1373-1376, 1965.

17. Clark HW, Bailey JS, Brown TMcP: New observations of mycoplasma infectivity and immunity. Fifth Interscience Conference of Antimicrobial Agents and Chemotherapy and IVth International Congress of Chemotherapy, Washington, DC, 1965.

18. Brown TMcP, Bailey JS, Felts WE, Clark HW: Mycoplasma antibodies in synovia. Arthritis Rheum. 9:495, 1966.

19. Fowler RC, Brown TMcP, Clark HW: Mycoplasmata and bacterial L-forms in rheumatoid diseases. In Proceedings of the Conference on the Relationship of Mycoplasma to Rheumatoid Arthritis and Related Disease, Decker J, ed. U.S. PHS Publication #1523, 1966.

20. Clark HW: Discussion of Mycoplasma immological problems. 2nd Congress on the Biology of Mycoplasmas. Ann. N.Y. Acad. Sci. 143:704-706, 1967.

21. Clark HW, Bailey JS, Brown TMcP: Variations in mycoplasma antigen activity. In Mycoplasma Diseases of Man. Sprossig M, Witzleb W, eds. Rheinhaardsbrunn Castle, VEB Gustov Fischer Verlag, Jena, Germany 1969.

22. Brown TMcP, Bailey JS, Clark HW, Gray CW, Clevenger AB, Heilen R.: Rheumatoid-type illness in gorilla with immunologic association of isolated mycoplasma and clinical remission following intravenous oxytetracycline therapy. 9th Interscience Conference on Antimicrobial Agents and Chemotherapy, 1969.

228

23. Brown TMcP, Bailey JS, Clark HW, Gray CW, Clevenger AB, Heilen R. Rheumatoid-type illness in gorilla with immunologic association of isolated mycoplasma and clinical remission following intravenous oxytetracycline therapy. Smithsonian Institution National Zoological Park, Annual Report, 1970.

24. Brown TMcP, Clark HW, Bailey JS, Gray CW: A mechanistic approach to treatment of rheumatoid-type arthritis naturally occurring in a gorilla. Trans. Am. Clin. Climatol. Assoc. 82:227-247, 1970.

25. Brown TMcP, Clark HW, Bailey JS: Relationship between mycoplasma antibodies and rheumatoid factors (RF). Arthritis Rheum. 13:309-310, 1970.

26. Clark HW, Bailey JS, Brown TMcP: Mycoplasma: Potential autoantigens? Xth International Congress for Microbiology, 92, 1970.

27. Clark HW, Bailey JS, Brown TMcP: Mycoplasma variations induced by penicillin. Bacteriol. Proceed., 1971.

28. Bailey JS, Clark HW, Brown TMcP: Characteristics of rabbit induced antibodies to human synovium and their relationship to mycoplasma. Am. Soc. Microbiol. Abstracts, M15, 82, 1972.

29. Clark HW, Brown TMcP: Association of mycoplasma antigens with vaccines from cell cultures. Am. Soc. Microbiol. Abstracts, M16, 82, 1972.

30. Clark HW, Bailey JS, Brown TMcP: Mycoplasma antigenic and immunogenic activity. Am. Soc. Microbiol. Abstracts, M35, 79, 1973.

31. Brown TMcP, Clark HW, Bailey JS: Mycoplasmas in pleural effusion of rheumatoid arthritis. XIIIth International Congress of Rheumatology, Japan, Abstract 594 in Excerpta Medica, 1973.

32. Brown TMcP, Clark HW, Bailey JS: Natural occurrence of rheumatoid arthritis in great apes —a new animal model. Proceedings of the Zoological Society of Philadelphia Centennial Symposium of Science and Research, 1974.

33. Bailey JS, Clark HW, Brown TMcP, Iden KI: Radial diffusion analysis of mycoplasma desoxyribonuclease. Am. Soc. Microbiol. 59, 1975.

34. Clark HW, Brown TMcP: Another look at mycoplasma. Arthritis Rheum. 19:649-650, 1976.

35. Clark HW, Bailey JS, Brown TMcP: Mycoplasma-hypersensitivity reactions. Proc. Soc. Gen. Microbiol. III 171, 1976.

36. Clark HW, Bailey JS, Brown TMcP: Mycoplasma-hypersensitivity in rheumatoid tissues. XIV International Congress of Rheumatology, Abstract #1107, 1977.

37. Brown TMcP, Clark HW, Boswell JT, Bailey JS. The essential role of the joint scan to assess basic therapeutic gain in rheumatoid arthritis. XIV International Congress of Rheumatology, Abstract #551, 137, 1977.

38. Clark HW: Guillain-Barre Syndrome. Letter Am. Soc. Microbiol. News 43(5):241, 1977.

39. Brown TMcP, Clark HW, Bailey JS, Gray CW: Rheumatoid-type arthritis naturally occurring in a gorilla—a three year follow-up report of a mechanistic approach to treatment. Proceedings of the XV International Symposium uber die Erkrankungen der Zootiere, Kolmarden, 1973.

40. Brown TMcP, Clark HW, Bailey JS: Rheumatoid arthritis in the gorilla: A study of mycoplasma-host interaction in pathogenesis and treatment. In Comparative Pathology of Zoo Animals. Montali RJ, Migaki G., eds. Smithsonian Institution Press, 1980.

41. Clark HW, Laughlin DC, Bailey JS, Brown TMcP: Mycoplasma species and arthritis in captive elephants. J. Zoo An. Med. 11:3-15, 1980.

42. Brown TMcP, Clark HW, Bailey JS, Attia MW. Comparative aspects of rheumatoid arthritis in the gorilla and man. International Congress of Rheumatology, 1981.

43. Attia MW, Clark HW, Brown TMcP: Evaluation of lymphocyte populations and their mitogenic activity in relation to serum copper and immunoglobulin levels in rheumatoid arthritis. Allergy 47(8):99-103, 1981.

44. Brown TMcP, Bailey JS, Iden KI, Clark HW: Antimycoplasma approach to the mechanism and the control of rheumatoid disease. In Inflammatory Diseases and Copper, Sorenson JRJ, ed. Humana Press, Clifton, N.J. 1982.

45. Attia MW, Clark HW, Brown TMcP, Ali MK, Bellanti JA. Inhibition of polymorphonu clear leukocyte migration by sera of patients with rheumatoid arthritis. Ann. Allergy 48:21-24, 1982.

46. Attia MW, Shams AJ, Ali MK, Land LW, Clark HW, Brown TMcP, Bellanti JA: Studies of phagocytic cell function in rheumatoid arthritis. I. Phagocytic and metabolic activities of neutrophils. Ann. Allergy 48:279-287, 1982.

47. Attia MW, Shams AJ, Ali MK, Land LW, Clark HW, Brown TMcP, Bellanti JA: Studies of phagocytic functions in rheumatoid arthritis. II. Effects of serum factors in phagocytic and metabolic activities of neutrophils. Ann. Allergy 48:266-270, 1982.

48. Clark HW, Bailey JS, Brown TMcP: Properties supporting the role of mycoplasmas in rheumatoid arthritis. Reviews of Infectious Diseases, Vol. 4: S238, 1982.

49. Clark HW, Brown TMcP: The antimycoplasma approach to the treatment of rheumatoid arthritis. Report to the U.S. House of Representatives Subcommittee for Appropriations, Hearings Part 9: 714-741, 1984.

50. Clark HW, Bailey JS, Brown TMcP: Medium-dependent properties of mycoplasmas. Diagn. Microbiol. Infect. Dis. 3: 283-294, 1985.

51. Bailey JS, Clark HW, Brown TMcP: SuperOxide as an agent of toxic potential for mycoplasmas. 85th Meeting of the ASM, 1985.

52. Brown TMcP, Hochberg MC, Hicks JT, Clark HW: Antibiotic therapy of rheumatoid arthritis: A retrospective cohort study of 98 patients with 451 patient-years of follow-up. XVIth International Congress of Rheumatology, Sydney, 1985.

53. Bailey JS, Clark HW, Brown TMcP: Profile of a mycoplasma isolate from rheumatoid synovium. 86th meeting of the ASM, 1986.

54. Clark HW, Coker-Vann MR, Bailey JS, Brown TMcP: Detection of mycoplasma antigens in immune complexes. International Organization for Mycoplasmology meeting, Birmingham, AL, 1986.

55. Clark HW: Mycoplasmal immune complexes - A perinatal pathogen? Ann. N.Y. Acad. Sci. 549: 222-224, 1988.

56. Clark HW, Coker-Vann MR, Bailey JS, Brown TMcP: Detection of mycoplasmas in immune complexes from rheumatoid arthritis synovial fluids. Ann. Allergy 60: 394-398, 1988.

57. Clark HW: Myoplasma bound IgG expresses autoantigenic anti-idiotypic antibodies. Am. Soc. Microbiol., 1989.

58. Clark HW: Papers #52 & #54. Symposium on Fertility in the Great Apes, Atlanta, GA, 1989.

59. Clark HW: Mycoplasma bound IgG expresses autoantigenic anti-idiotypic antibodies. XVIIth ILAR Congress of Rheumatology, 771, 1989.

60. Clark HW: The potential role of mycoplasma as autoantigens and immune complexes in chronic vascular pathogenesis. Am. V. Primatol. 24: 235-243, 1991.

61. Clark HW: Rheumatoid arthritis. In Medical Management of the Elephant, Mikota SK, Sargent EL, Ranglack GS, Indira publ. 151-157, 1994.

62. Clark HW Tetracycline correction. Letter to the Editor, Ann. 123:393, 1995.

63. Clark HW: Mycoplasmas and disease. Letter in ASM News. 62:617, 1996.

Index

collagenase, 54, 81, 83, 101, 106, 110, 111, 112, 149, 154, 155, 165, 179, 180, 189

collagen vascular disorders, 108, 110, 111, 191

Congress (see U.S. Senate and U.S. House of Representatives, 27, 48, 50, 54, 55, 57, 60, 61, 62, 65-68, 92, 93, 95-98, 126, 127, 129, 131, 134, 154, 157, 160-163, 165, 173, 175, 176, 181, 183, 184, 187, 189, 193, 194

connective tissue, 16, 44, 73, 83, 110, 111, 154, 155

copper, 45, 46, 82- 84, 92, 94, 95, 101, 109, 117, 131, 141, 153, 156

copper bracelet, 94, 95

cortisone, 27, 41, 44, 85, 105, 166, 194, 198

cost of arthritis, 9, 57, 95, 125, 250

Cousins, Norman, 73

Cranston, Senator, 54

cyclophosphamide, 86, 92

cyclosporine, 88, 92

D

Decker, John, 129, 154

degenerative joint disease, 3, 6

dental, 44, 107, 111, 154, 179, 181, 183

Department of Health, Education, & Welfare (DHEW), 19, 55

Department of Health & Human Services (DHHS), 19

Department of Vocational Rehabilitation (DVR), 19

depression, 73, 157

diabetes, 47, 88, 110, 111, 137, 138, 168, 179, 183, 190-193, 195, 196

diagnosis, differential, 35, 148, 150, 151, 156, 196

Dienes, Lewis, 26, 27, 89

diet, 20, 25, 46, 79-81, 84, 103, 195

digestive enzymes, 53, 54

disability benefits (see Social Security), 97, 184

disease modifying anti-rheumatic drugs (DMARD), 83, 85, 92, 105

dogs, 34, 39, 41

drugs, 28, 35, 40, 64, 67, 79, 82-88, 91-93, 95, 100, 101, 104-106, 108, 112, 113, 117, 121, 122-126, 128, 129, 132, 133, 140, 146, 148, 150, 153, 157-158, 160, 173, 174, 176, 189, 190

E

Eaton agent, 28, 91

Egypt, 14, 74

elderly, 23, 24, 44

elephants, 22, 34, 39, 42, 93, 166, 187

emotional effects, 90

Epstein-Barr virus (EBV), 67

erythromycin, 87, 88, 132, 141, 146, 189

Excerpta Medica Index, 62, 148

exercise, 20, 35, 45, 77-79, 112, 174, 195

F

families, 32, 184

fatigue, 23, 24, 45, 77, 78, 138, 157, 194, 196

fever, 15, 40, 48, 58, 81, 102

financial problems, 31, 160, 173, 182, 191

Finland, 59, 145, 146

FK 506, 87, 88, 189, 190

Fossey, Diane, 34, 37

Fox, H., 34, 35, 37

G

gamma globulin, 16, 68, 90, 106, 167, 191

Geigy Pharmaceuticals, 93

genetics, 25, 33, 46, 172, 177

genito-urinary tract, 27, 28, 48, 62, 107, 116, 155

George Washington University, 35, 197

gold salts, 16, 26, 27, 48, 67, 84, 85, 105, 106, 122, 123, 125, 128, 133, 141, 146, 147, 166

gorillas-great apes, (see Tomoka), 34, 35, 36, 37, 39, 40, 52, 53, 74, 93, 96, 97, 98, 99, 102, 122, 123, 130, 142, 148, 166, 187

gout, 14, 44, 46

Graft vs Host reaction, 87, 190

H

Hartford Foundation, John A., 50

Harvard Medical Center, 89

hate, 23, 61, 73, 137, 177

health insurance, 192

Healy, Bernadine, 177

heat therapy, 77

Heberden. William, 14

hemoglobin, 82

235

236

Note: To obtain further information about the treatment and infectious etiology of rheumatoid diseases, send your request with a large self-addressed envelope and $.64 postage to:

The Road Back Foundation
4985 North Lake Hill Road
Delaware, Ohio 43015-9249

For additional copies of *Why Arthritis?* send a check or money order (U.S. funds) for $18.95 per copy plus shipping fee of $3.00 for U.S.A. to:

Mycoplasma Research Institute
P.O. Box 640040
Beverly Hills, FL 34464-0040